PSYCHIATRY BETWEEN THE WARS, 1918-1945

Contributions in Medical History
Series Editor: John Burnham

Women & Men Midwives
Medicine, Morality, and Misogyny in Early America
Jane B. Donegan

American Midwives 1860 to the Present
Judy Barrett Litoff

Speech and Speech Disorders in Western Thought
Before 1600
Ynez Violé O'Neill

Sex, Diet, and Debility in Jacksonian America:
Sylvester Graham and Health Reform
Stephen Nissenbaum

Shock, Physiological Surgery, and George Washington Crile:
Medical Innovation in the Progressive Era
Peter C. English

Professionalizing Modern Medicine: Paris Surgeons and
Medical Science and Institutions in the 18th Century
Toby Gelfand

Medicine and Its Technology: An Introduction to
the History of Medical Instrumentation
Audrey B. Davis

In Her Own Words: Oral Histories of Women Physicians
*Regina Markell Morantz, Cynthia Stodola Pomerleau, and
Carol Hansen Fenichel, editors*

Technicians of the Finite: The Rise and Decline of the
Schizophrenic in American Thought, 1840-1960
S. P. Fullinwider

PSYCHIATRY BETWEEN THE WARS, 1918-1945

A Recollection

Walter Bromberg

Contributions in Medical History, Number 10

GREENWOOD PRESS
Westport, Connecticut • London, England

Library of Congress Cataloging in Publication Data

Bromberg, Walter, 1900-
  Psychiatry between the wars, 1918-1945.

  (Contributions in medical history, ISSN 0147-1058;
no. 10)
  Bibliography: p.
  Includes index.
  1. Psychiatry—United States—History.   2. Psychiatry
—New York (N.Y.)—History.   3. Neuropsychiatry—United
States—History.   I. Title.   II. Series.
RC 339.A1B76   616.89'00973   82-6153
ISBN 0-313-23460-4 (lib. bdg.)   AACR2

Library of Congress Catalog Card Number: 82-6153
ISBN: 0-313-23460-4
ISSN: 0147-1058

First published in 1982

Greenwood Press
A division of Congressional Information Service, Inc.
88 Post Road West, Westport, Connecticut 06881

Printed in the United States of America

10 9 8 7 6 5 4 3 2 1

To
Joan, David, and Mark
How it was in the "Old Days"

If you can talk with crowds and keep your virtue,
Or walk with Kings—nor lose the common touch.

Kipling

CONTENTS

SERIES FOREWORD

Occasionally in medicine a particular individual will make out-standing contributions to the profession and also will have the perspective to write a broad history that makes sense of the past and guides successor historians and young colleagues in under-standing the problems that confront practitioner and researcher alike. Such a person is Walter Bromberg, M.D., a truly eminent American psychiatrist and the author of a historical classic in the field, *Man Above Humanity, A History of Psychotherapy,* which first appeared in 1937 under the title, *The Mind of Man.*

In the work here, Dr. Bromberg offers a combination of historical perspective and personal recollection of psychiatric history as he has experienced it in his own life, focusing on the years from World War I to World War II. Those were great days for what was called "neuropsychiatry." Dr. Bromberg not only portrays them but suggests the power of the scientific and historical forces that swayed those who lived through these decades. He follows the way psychiatry appeared in the journals that professionals read, and he weaves in his experiences with some of the most exciting figures in an exciting field. People who care about mental health, or just a good story, will gain from this book a unique sense of how clinical neurology inspired members of a generation who then turned with enthusiasm to both psychoanalyis and physiological therapies.

In his personal introduction the author sketches some of the important elements in the sociocultural climate before World War I that set the stage for the great changes that occurred in the way the mind and its problems were popularly conceived. During the fluid years that followed, from 1918 to 1945, groundwork was laid for the subsequent spectacular post-World War II expansion of American psychiatry when the "shrink" became established as a major element in American society. In his thoughtful narrative Dr. Bromberg combines social matrix with the inside story as he saw it and shows how the culture as well as the profession developed the potentiality for the explosive growth of psychiatry that came after 1945.

PREFACE

The period between World War I and World War II witnessed the accelerated growth of psychiatry in the United States. Although some have perceived psychiatry as a "fresh new specialty" that arose after 1945, as Melvin Sabshin has pointed out, its history antedates the wars by several centuries.[1] This book is limited to a small segment of that history; with due regard for our debt to pre-World War I neurology and psychiatry from Germany, England, France, and Vienna, it concerns American accomplishments. More specifically, the material presented here is restricted to activities on the East Coast, particularly New York City, for New York virtually formed the epicenter of neuropsychiatric happenings during this period. The author was witness to, and involved in, many of these happenings. This book, therefore, is history-as-experienced and hence may include a personal bias in the events that have been selected as significant and in personalities presented.

Another factor must be noted from which all personal histories suffer, aside from the fiction of "total recall." This is the inescapable factual incompleteness that was expressed by Louis Gottschalk, professor of history at the University of Chicago, when he wrote:

Only a part of what was observed in the past was remembered . . . only a part of what was remembered was recorded . . . only a part of what survived . . . is credible.
History as told . . . is only the historian's expressed part of the understood part of the credible part of the discovered part of history-as recorded.[2]

The book itself grew out of a "living history" tape recording made at the Library of the American Psychiatric Association in Washington, D.C., in November of 1977 at the invitation of Dr. Roger Watson and Jean Jones, who were the interviewers. The tape became the property of the library archives. The somewhat chaotic recollections then placed on tape have been enlarged and reorganized here to ensure a more cohesive whole. This enlargement was deemed important because the development of psychiatry between 1918 and 1945 rivaled that of any comparable period of medical history. My thanks are offered to Dr. Watson and Ms. Jones for their invitation to engage in this association function.

Particularly valuable criticism was given to the draft of the manuscript by George Mora, M.D., a research associate in the history of medicine at Yale University and by Jacques Quen, M.D., a member of the section on psychiatric history at Cornell University Medical Center. The expert critique given the manuscript by John Burnham, series editor for Greenwood Press, professor of history at Ohio State University, and a distinguished psychiatric historian, was invaluable. The librarians at the Sacramento Medical Society, the University of California at Davis Medical Center, and the California State Library, helped to fill some of the gaps in my memory and helped to check the references. I wish to thank my secretary, Diane Baetge, who laboriously typed and retyped the drafts of the manuscript.

Finally, I wish to express my gratitude to those teachers and associates now assigned to the psychiatric section of a medical Valhalla, where it is presumed they may eternally ponder the vagaries of the human mind.

Walter Bromberg, M.D.

NOTES

1. Melvin Sabshin, Editorial Comment, *Journal of Clinical Psychiatry* 40 (March 1979):112.

2. Louis Gottschalk, *Understanding History: A Primer of Historical Method* (New York: A. A. Knopf, 1950), p. 46.

A PERSONAL INTRODUCTION

Americans born after 1929 may find it difficult to envision the life-styles, social values, and attitudes of urban dwellers in the early days of this century. Since this book is, in part, a recollective account of American psychiatry between the two world wars, it may be illuminating before the story is unfolded to provide a glimpse of some of the life routines at the turn of the century from a boy's stance, for in the last analysis society and psychiatry are profoundly related.

For myself, I was born in Manhattan, in the Tompkins Square area, which was peopled mostly by immigrant Poles, Russians, and other Slavic stock. There my mother and father, intent on becoming Americanized in the shortest possible time, slaved to learn English and avoided Russian except to converse on privy matters. The intelligentsia who crowded the Tenth Street and Avenue A area lived in rat-infested tenements, but they enjoyed the freedom to discuss over copious glasses of "chy" (tea) the endless problems of European politics.

A few years after my parents' arrival in the New World in 1893, Father, who had been apprenticed to a jeweler in Moscow, managed to earn enough on Rivington Street to escape the brick and mortar snake pits of the East Side. Intent on moving to Brooklyn to be "close to nature," my family first landed in Brownsville, then in the lower reaches of Park Slope, and finally on the crest of the ridge that ran through Brooklyn from the Narrows to eastern Long Island. Our home lay in a semirural area bordering on Prospect Park, where venerable trees caused Father to exclaim: "A dream, just like the birch forests around Moscow."

Because Mother was a romantic, she named my oldest brother, born in 1894, for Edward VII of England; my sister, Sophie, born in 1897, for Sophia, Queen of the Bulgars; and I, for Sir Walter Scott; my second brother, born in 1902, was named for Julius Caesar; and the youngest, (not yet on the scene) Lester, received his name from the suggestion of a nurse who hailed from Michigan, which Mother thought represented America in essence. In an early thrust toward Americanization, Father's name, Zachary (zaxap), was precipitiously changed to George. None of us received middle names, although the midwife who delivered me added an "N" (presumably for Nathan but never spelled out) to the birth certificate in a pang of conscience at this rapid Anglicization.

Our move to the crest of Brooklyn, not seventy yards from Prospect Park, opened a new era for us. The hub of the neighborhood was a quadrangle anchored on its four corners by a grocer, a dry-goods store, an ice cream parlor, which was soon to be replaced by a barbershop, and the ubiquitous McCauley's Bar. Each of these commerical enterprises contributed its own special flavor. the grocer, a Mr. Christenson, a rotund man who sold broken crackers at a discount and cut chunks of butter from a wooden tub with a long knife that was wielded with the precision of a toolmaker, spent his days in knowledgeable disorder. Being sent to the store was an experience in viewing affluence; there were barrels of pickles, cases of crackers, tins of coffee and tea, a large-wheeled coffee grinder, mounds of bread, bundles of kindling wood tied with wispy hemp, slices of ham, baloney, and bacon (all cut by hand) a wooden tray of "greens" and eggs, and rolls of oiled paper. Mr. Christenson ran his store informally. Whether one ordered half a loaf of bread, ten cents worth of "broken crackers," or "a shilling's worth of yeggs" (the Irish still spoke in terms of shillings and pence), his cheerfulness neither diminished nor augmented. The dry-goods store across the street, which was operated by two maiden ladies, the Misses Mason and Lockwood, similarly shared this quintessence of benevolent commerce. The "girls," eternally smiling, sold collar buttons, Clarks thread, ruching by the yard, linen and celluloid collars, and cotton cloth that was measured between two immutable brass buttons on the counter.

The diversity of nations and religions could not have been better arranged to illustrate the American melting pot theory. The neighborhood represented a combination of strivers and amblers, of workers and drifters, of kerosene lamps and electric lights, of hard-coal furnaces and pot-bellied stoves. It struggled between country and city in time as well as in physical extension. The city lamplighter, riding on his bicycle, lit the street gaslights at twilight with his magic wand, while the small, frame houses picked up their reflections in their own glass-chimneyed lamps. The bandy-legged postman, a bag slung over his shoulder, made his rounds, while mothers sent little notes to other mothers through the agency of racing boys. As the area filled with new dwellings, the older houses shrank within the shadow of brick and granite city houses. The lots filled in; modern homes became standard; bright, well-fed Jewish children swelled the school enrollment; the street jangled with the noise of play, and "rus" bowed to "urb."

For the boy of the time, the streets offered such entrancing spectacles as open and closed trolley cars, where the motormen, encased in their throne rooms (the front platforms) were the unchallenged masters of the street. When they "danged" their gongs, few truck drivers or pedestrians questioned their right of way. The motorman was master of the vessel, the conductor was his majordomo and the passengers his subject.

While trolleys were power incarnate, horse-drawn wagons ran the gamut from delicacy to ponderousness. Wagons emblazoned with bucolic scenes—a pheasant in full color, a spanking colt in flight, a white cow grazing in a meadow—were of the daintier breed. The trucks, however, were more prosaic and stated their business boldly—ICE or COAL or EXPRESS. The closer to essential industry, the simpler the legend. Horses were fascinating too. The fearless steeds that thundered before fire engines on lifesaving runs differed from mousy, swaybacked hacks that pulled the junkman's wagon through the streets.

Excitement on the streets was counterbalanced by familiar drudgery at home. Our moral teachings, excluding Sunday school instruction, involved food as much as the Decalogue. Mother, a devotee of Dr. Elmer Lee, a leading advocate of brown sugar and graham bread and a crusader against foods artificially colored with aniline dyes, warned us against meat that looked fresh but derived its pinkness from the deadly preservative, benzoate of soda. It was clear to her that those who colored foods, especially candy, were embarked on a fiendish program to destroy children's bones and teeth. The *Index Expurgatorium* listed the marvels of various candies—"Uncle Sam" bars, a wonderful combination of chocolate and nuts; pastel-shaded bars of marshmallow; lemon drops; taffy; sheets of white paper dotted by little dabs of pink, violet, white, and blue candies that when pulled off carried fringes of paper; and peppermint discs with printed words. Mother seemed overjoyed that Dr. Harvey Wiley of pure food fame had uncovered a subversive plot to undermine the health of American children that could be countered by such allowable confections as licorice and rock candy.

The real danger, according to Mother, especially to girls, lay in yielding to John Barleycorn. One sure entrance to this future life of hell lay through the ladies' entrance of the corner saloon, popularly known as the "side door." The ladies' entrance was graced provacatively by a glass door embossed with lillies and roses blowing delicately in the wind and tinted pink or amber, which effectively hid happenings inside. A girl entering a saloon with an untried escort could be given a "knockout drop" and dragged semiconscious upstairs to be deflowered in a dank room.

Prohibitions against alcohol spread to the tragedy of smoking. The smoking of corn tassles wrapped in newspaper, barely known to anxious mothers, ceded to the real danger of Sweet Caporals, Meccas, Cleo's, or even the straw-tipped Melachrinos, which an esthetic uncle occasionally left in plain view during his Sunday visits to our home. Smoking butts left by adults in our clubhouse cave was an accepted experiment in sinfulness, but acquisition of the habit was anathema. Teachers and mothers united in deploring the stunting effects of tobacco, the "filthy weed." For proof they pointed to the emaciated man who was exhibited at the Coney Island sideshow and billed as a "Slave to Tobacco." His waddling gait and gaunt frame with unbelievably thin shanks and arms sent shivers down the spines of all who saw him—the ultimate in physical deterioration. Smoking like a chimney while on exhibition, the "freak" pleaded with his audience to save themselves from a fate worse than death by eschewing tobacco. Much later

I learned that he was an advanced case of muscular dystrophy, foisted on the public as a victim of the tobacco habit. Of this I knew nothing at the time, and our conferences in the cave yielded no light on the subject. Yet the romance of smoking transcended all homely, lifesaving advice. How could cigarette packages carrying pictures of baseball heroes, Indian scouts, and American generals contain such fearsome threats to American youth?

Other sources of immorality faced Brooklyn mothers. There were the "nickelodeons" (named for their admission charge of five cents), small auditoriums that were built by disemboweling saloons and installing seats on the floor and a white screen on the wall on which the moving images were projected. A suspicion of illicitness hung over the nickelodeon, a heritage from its relation to the penny arcades, where men gloated over a series of flipped picture cards that showed women removing petticoats and corsets. Leaders in the community declaimed against them, and a Chicago judge in 1907 expressed his horror forcefully: "Those nickelodeons indirectly or directly caused more juvenile crimes . . . than all other causes combined."

Public schools of the 1904-1914 period also reeked of the spirit of absolutism. Going to school represented a fixed element in life that was interrupted only by vacations—Easter, Thanksgiving, Christmas, and summer. It was also interrupted by scarlet fever, pneumonia and diphtheria. Sometimes children dropped out of school when orphaned, but the orphanage immediately picked up the scholastic threads; there was no escape until one reached the distant eventuality of his or her fourteenth year. Until then school ground on, oblivious of the adult world, supported on the tripod of "Effort," "Achievement," and "Deportment." For its pupils it meant memorizing, copying, and learning under the control of persons bent on making life unpleasant "for your own good."

Teachers believed in two fundamental propositions: the immutability of facts and the importance of drills. In history it was dates; in geography, boundaries of the various countries; in mathematics, mental arithmetic. Besides the mind-improvement aspects of such exercises, practical applications lurked in the background. How else could one foil an unscrupulous storekeeper? The uses of an alert mind were endless! Mental arithmetic contained a magic of its own, second only to fact accumulation; mountains of facts like measuring units—the bushel, peck, hogshead, troy and avoirdupois weight, pennyweight, dram, ounces, foot, ell, hand, fathom. In a soft moment the teacher implied that it was true that someday these ancient units would fall before the onslaught of the metric system. Meanwhile, "now is the time to learn when your mind is impressionable. Do you want to be a hod carrier?" There was no retort to such impressive dogma. The fate of hod carrier or day laborer brought shudders; it was a disgrace equal only to conviction for larceny or murder.

From our side of the educational wall, respect for facts became entrenched. When the charts picturing the countries of Europe (or states of the Union) announced that Sardinia was deep purple, Switzerland, pale pink, France, a vivid red, or New York and New Jersey, green and salmon respectively, or when the text proclaimed that Spain exported cork, olive oil, and wines, who could rob us of this intellectual possession? A gain was a gain, and rote made it yours forever. Still we sensed that our teachers were a dedicated lot as they moved beyond facts to ethics, to principles of the "good life," stories of virtue, honesty, and hard work.

The devout, even ascetic influences of our principal and teachers were emphasized at weekly assemblies. Here the pupils would march into the auditorium to the tune of "Stars and Stripes Forever" to face the principal who stood before the Corinthian columns that graced the rear of the platform. This stirring music pounded out on the piano by Miss Seidenberg, a tiny, serious-faced teacher from the seventh grade, set the tone. Then the principal, Miss Laing, a dignified gray-haired woman, would read the Psalms, usually the twenty-third, with a sense of infinite faith that she was implanting eternal verities in young minds. Afterwards the assistant principal would take over, introducing one of the pupils who would recite a poem or tell a brief story rehearsed for the occasion. A girl attired in a white dress or a boy in a white shirt would mount the platform, make a slight bow, rattle off the verse, and depart from the stage like a frightened deer. Assembly concluded with Miss Seidenberg again thundering out on the piano the "Stars and Stripes Forever." We would march out of the auditorium uplifted and inspired. But Miss Laing's charism did not last long. As we left the schoolhouse, we plunged back into our universe of roughhouse, pubertal play, and sexually tinged pranks; juvenile hellions in the tradition of *Lord of the Files.*

At home schooling was of a different sort. In contrast to Miss Laing's subtle but gentle sermonizing, I often encountered Mother and Mrs. Budinoff, a neighbor, chatting endlessly in the kitchen over glasses of tea. They spoke of "advanced thinkers" like John Most, Emma Goldman, and Alexander Berkman. Apparently John Most, an anarchist who had been expelled from Germany, was scheduled to speak in New York. This exciting event coincided with the arrival of a small magazine titled *Mother Earth.* Both women discussed it avidly, including the relationship between Berkman and Emma Goldman who went in and out of prison for arguing too much in public and for believing in free love, which meant to me that the man and woman had different names. From the talk around the kitchen table, I supposed that anarchism was fun because those who espoused it didn't seem to work much. It also meant that you made fun of the judges and police and hypocrites who gave their money to churches but suppressed the masses all week.

The romantic view of revolution gathered from Mother and Mrs. Budinoff's tea talks was split assunder by revelations from Uncle Sol, a civil engineer turned IWW, concerning the brutality of time spent in jail contrasted with the flowing conversation of the intelligentsia; Kropotkin and Pushkin were replaced with talk about "scabs" and "Pinkertons."

In contrast to this striving for freedom of expression among adults, in our neighborhood at least and undoubtedly elsewhere, a curious series of phobias and counterphobias invaded children's play. If you stepped on a crack in the sidewalk, your mother would die; if you stepped on an ant, a downpour would result; if you wanted to share a pal's candy, apple, or bicycle ride, you yelled "dibs." The countercharm, "ackie," if shouted before the claim of "dibs" was heard, foreclosed all future claims. The estoppel "fins," made by crossing the middle finger over the index finger, conferred protection from injury or failure; it could itself be rendered innocuous by uttering the word "everies." Sometimes, to evade the effect of the countercharm, you made the sign of "fins" unseen in your pockets, in which case you had priority and all contingencies were covered. The charms and countercharms represented immutable laws from which there was no appeal.

Our allegiance to convention was reflected in odd ways. During the baseball season, one had to be "for" a team, and once locked into that brotherhood there was no retreat. To the question "Who are you for?" you answered, the Giants, Dodgers, or Yanks; once the choice was made, you remained among the faithful—win, lose, or draw.

There were other unwritten laws in our society that further bound us in ironclad conformity. A younger brother was to be protected at all costs from physical abuse and a mother to be shielded from hearing about misfortunes, although she had an uncanny ability to divine the truth immediately on sighting the nontalebearer. The rule states that whatever went wrong—a broken window, an arrest by a cop, a fight in which blood flowed— was to be concealed from Mama. Later Pop could hear the ugly truth, and in the calm atmosphere of judicial decision the miscreant could be whipped with a belt, let off with a reprimand, or taken to the station house for a friendly conversation with the desk sergeant. This man-to-man stuff could be faced openly, especially since it was acknowledged by the parent that "it happened to me once," a revelation that made the whole world kin.

Other dangers beset us in play: pulled muscles, gnarled knuckles, and that mysterious condition known as "rupture." This curious condition in older men, signalized by a bulge in the groin, carried a sexual connotation: a man had to be careful of his genital area. Stradling a fence or even a rope was known to have caused ruptures. It was obvious that athleticism was not without its dangers. Interest among us in disease was both perennial and obsessional. It ranged from warnings that if you played with yourself, "it" might fall off or rot away to unattended scratches on the skin that would unquestionably result in blood poisoning.

Talk of disease was ubiquitous; measles, scarlet fever, diphtheria, and the recently discovered appendicitis were the prime concerns of mothers and the main substance of their conversation within our hearing. The controversy surrounding the replacement of regular high shoes with Oxfords (called "half-shoes") became grist to our clinical mill. How could a laboring man find support for his ankles in these newfangled Oxfords? And where would one find room in half-shoes for arch supporters, the newly discovered remedy for the newly discovered disease called "flat feet"?

From general advice preachments went to particulars of behavior such as in the command, "take your hands out of your pockets!" To this misuse of hands was added even more stringent proscriptions against spitting. For men and boys spitting on the sidewalk seemed a natural function whose cause, a condition known as "catarrh," afflicted almost everybody. Remedies for catarrh were legion, but the simplest method for the expulsion of mucus from the nose and throat appeared to be spitting. For the average male, spitting was au naturel. Dickens in his American travel book in the 1840s remarked on thick clots of mucus, dried and fresh, that he saw openly displayed in hotels, bars, and on the streets of old Gotham.

Sex vied with baseball as the arcanum of masculinity. One of our mentors, Doc Smith, a medical student who big-brothered us on many a summer afternoon, plunged us into the center of life, which for him meant female anatomy. Doc, a friendly man whose close-clipped hair and hawk nose projected a professional air, let it be known that he preferred to be known as Doc rather than Doctor, a preference I thought showed true democracy but turned out to rest on his having been flunked out of Long Island Medical College. Dock Smith loved his audience; the more we hovered over him and lowered our voices to escape being overheard by the girls, the more luridly he slanted his stories. These dealt with venereal diseases—"syph" and "clap"—accompanied with pencil sketches of anatomical and pathological details.

If the vagaries of the sexual impulse were never openly discussed by parents, matters of hygiene and illness were never slighted. Almost any mother, and certainly every grandmother, could diagnose measles and the fever. Visits to the local physician were limited to emergencies when blood had been spilled or to confirm a maternal diagnosis of scarlet fever or diphtheria. Obscure matters like childbirth and miscarriage involved doctors, but midwives still were high up on the consultation panel. For more complex illnesses or chronic maladies that did not seem to clear up with commonsense remedies, a visit to Manhattan for a consultation with a specialist was justified.

At home, medical matters followed a more modern course. Because Mother had graduated from the Nurse's Training School at the University of Moscow, she was wary of pallid American doctors, youthful and beardless, with little knowledge of European medicine. However, when Mother discovered that the pages of *Health,* edited by Dr. Charles A. Tyrell and Dr. Elmer Lee, advocated the cause of brown sugar, brown rice, and other vitamin-rich foods, she embraced the new gospel with enthusiasm. Prune juice, orange juice, and spinach water became the fluid road to health. As the authoritative Drs. Tyrell and Lee stated in their journal, there were evil side effects to "refined" foods:

A wrong diet is the chief cause of abnormal sexuality. Too stimulating foods excite the nerves . . . then the nerves control man instead of the man controlling the nerves . . . sex pleasures and immorality result from stimulation. . . . Stimulation is inflammation.

This sort of heretical talk from physicians ran counter to food practices in our community. In the first place, everyone knew that lettuce, carrots, and spinach were "rabbit food," that men who labored needed their beer, that women were satisfied with tea, and that children grew fat on cereals and milk. Housewives protected their children from red meats; they kept stomachs "sweet" by insisting on wholesome foods; they purified the blood of their offspring with sulphur and molasses and irrigated the intestinal tract with Fletcher's Castoria. But no housewife would tinker with the "meat and potatoes" diet of working husbands, and few could see any harm in a piece of baloney on bread spread with lard for breakfast.

To spinach water and brown sugar, Mother added a new panacea—dried bread. In fact, an entire mythology grew up around fresh bread, especially hot bread or rolls, that stated these foodstuffs caused biliousness, heartburn, and waterbrash, conditions that alone were discomforting enough but when combined into the disease called "dyspepsia," spelled invalidism. To counteract this, stale or dry bread was recommended and reached its ultimate elegance in zweiback. Zweiback and milk were the avowed enemies of "weak, sour and upset" stomachs. If these dreaded conditions did not yield to this combination, the last recourse was to seltzer water, which was thought to be invincible because of its relation to the spas of Europe.

Besides rituals regarding foods, other formal customs among our neighbors were observed. Sunday was a special day, a colorful node in the monotonous grayness of the week. By common consent, working people slept late; youths slept into the afternoon, thus advertising their Saturday night carousing. Churchgoers in our area, mainly Roman Catholics, moved almost in a body with an obvious sense of righteousness to the Holy Name Church; Protestants filled their churches with a more subdued pride.

For ourselves we had no contact with the synagogue. Yiddish was considered a barbarism; the high holy days were noted only casually. Although an undeniable kinship grew in us toward the increasing number of Jews in the neighborhood, all my brothers and I were Bar Mitzvah drop-outs. Still, it occasioned no surprise later when we slid into the Jewish group in the community without obvious preparation. At the time, my interest was more closely tied to action than to religious concerns. That action was high school, where another world unfolded.

For the emerging adolescent, graduation from grammar school was epochal, an end to childhood. The choices were limited—high school or the securing of "working papers" and the subsequent "settling down," which ran a well-defined course. It meant working in a trade with one's father or family friend, or apprenticing oneself to a journeyman, and emerging one day several years later wheeling a baby carriage on the avenue with the fatuous smile of a young husband. The approved sequence—a trade or job in business, marrying early, "saving for a family"—held for all but a few who might escape the doom of regularity by a free-wheeling year out West or at sea, or "on the bum." Sooner or later the harness of regularity engulfed even the free soul, and its promise of "making good" turned into a rigid steel cage.

The image of high school contributed by my older brother sounded intriguing—Gallic wars, "veni, vidi, vinci," algebra, "student organizations," chess clubs, and football! The image blurred when I found out I was assigned to Manual Training High School, a name that dissipated the clouds of glory surrounding schools like Boy's High School and Erasmus Hall High School. We had been tricked, we thought: a trade school, just a cut above the obviously commercial Commercial High School! But reports kept seeping through that "Manual" did not deserve the condescension with which students destined for academic schools viewed it.

In fact the manual crafts were slipped in between regular subjects. Mr. Mueller, our German instructor, a stocky man equipped with a Prussian haircut and a military bearing, handled us like a company of raw recruits. The drudgery of declensions, of "der, die, das, dem, den," came to embody the precision of a field drill. Conjugations, tenses, genders, and cases fell into line under the whiplash of the drill master. His manners epitomized the highest of the Teutonic heavens, where "Hoch Deutsch" vanquished "Platt Deutsch," where "sitzfleish" (diligence) was a most valued asset, and the banner that floated overhead read "Arbeit macht das Leben Süss (work makes life sweet).

Each teacher was an adventure in individuality. Mr. Bates of the English department wore a wing collar, spoke in precise English, and held his book high under his armpit in the manner of a scholar; a Miss Batchelder who taught French reminded me more of "Hail Britannica" than of a petite Frenchwoman; Dr. Giovanni, whose prestige was enhanced by the fact that he taught Spanish, then hailed as the "coming language," was a florid, squarely built Italian who headed the Romance language department. School ground on until summer vacation arrived in middle June.

While Memorial Day was dedicated to war veterans and parades, the Fourth of July belonged to the glaring sun and Coney Island. No nonsessile Brooklynite neglected Coney Island at this pivotal point in summer. Except for a few timid oldsters and fashionable ladies who equipped themselves with parasols, the Fourth of July opened the sunburn season. We bared ourselves to the hot July sun at the beach, content to complain of pain and burning shoulders. The macerated peeling skin offered a delayed masochistic pleasure. Being burned by the sun was a badge of fortitude, for white skin was the order of the day. No one thought of gradually tanning themselves with chemical aids or sunbaths.

However, I was ready for more gritty experiences. Summertime jobs were not scarce for schoolboys. I answered an advertisement for messenger boys and found myself in a group of about fifteen at the entrance of an ancient building on Vesey Street in Manhattan. The area smelled of 1890; the solid buildings were decorated with ornate cornices, the streets were filled with trucks, and aproned drivers and helpers yelled, cursed, pulled boxes and unloaded merchandise in orderly confusion. A block away the Washington Market added to the noise and confusion. The shops on Church Street crowded each other, selling hardware, garden supplies, plants, clothes, shoes, and food to the crowds of commuters that passed toward the New Jersey ferries daily. The work was easy since the proprietor hired more schoolboys than he needed, presumably out of warm feelings as a benefactor of youth. He turned the task of managing the boys to his shipping clerk. The clerk, a slim, harried man who wore a green eyeshade and sleeve garters, carried the responsibilities of the business on his sloping shoulders. His tired voice clucked over us messengers like a sergeant's over a platoon of raw recruits.

As the summer wore on, the shipping clerk's relationship with us became more fraternal than paternal. He began to lift up the corners of his career as if to indicate that invoices, packages, deliveries, and stockroom cares only filled a part of his life. He confided his amorous adventures; how a Polish landlady pushed her husband out of the bedroom in his favor because he paid a dollar a month more than the other boarders. As he related the benefits of the single life in a realm of willing landladies, his tired blue eyes shone and his stooped shoulders were transformed into a bundle of eager muscles. Among ourselves we never doubted his Casanova-like adventures, his delineation of big-breasted from flat-chested women, his preference for Polish women, his assurance that every woman has her moment, if only you are there at the right time. Inwardly each of the delivery boys dredged up his own inexperience to compare in shame with that of our teacher. The shipping clerk stood as an authority on erotica; his advice was direct and specific. "Watch out for them streetwalkers," he would

say with a knowing wink. "Get a nice clean girl . . . but you
kids have a long way to go." Then he would launch into a long
recital, "Once when I was a young feller in Baltimore, I had this
woman . . ."

A shipping clerk was a vital part of most mercantile establish-
ments. In well-established firms he represented an analogue of
the faithful servant whose long service in a home had imprinted on
his soul the seal and form of the establishment. He would never
rise to the executive level nor would he ever sink. The shipping
clerk, the teamster, and the delivery boys (as long as they remained
there), all dwelt in a secure subterranean section of the mansion
of business. The boss's son lived on another level parallel to the
college graduate who entered the firm and was guaranteed to
succeed by virtue of a coating of knowledge that the boss did not
understand but bowed to nevertheless. The shipping clerk and his
boys were the troops, they the officers. I began to appreciate
the intertwining relationship between college and the strange world
of commerce.

In company with my brothers I became enmeshed in another
area of learning during my pre-high-school days. My mother heard
of open meetings of the Brooklyn Philosophical Society on Sundays
in a schoolhouse in Williamsburg. She attended a meeting and
came home with a surge of enthusiasm. For a year we accompanied
her to this Mecca of the mind. Sitting on the hard benches I heard
a series of new words—single tax, evolution, Darwinism—and new
names—Henry George, Huxley, Spencer. The words and names
were meaningless, but the clots of phrases have echoed down
the years to acquire significance in retrospect. If brother Jules and
I listened in a state of somnolence, enough engrams formed to
make socialism and the conflicts of evolution versus religion,
Darwinism versus the Bible, something of a reality later on. The
audience and Mother were enthralled by the discussion, especially
on that milestone Sunday when Emma Goldman held forth on the
platform for a full hour.

It was the speakers themselves that left a clearer impression on
me, notably a redheaded Irish socialist with a thick brogue, a
German named Theodore Schroeder who appeared to be a leader
because no one moved when he spoke, and two Jewish lawyers

named Morris Hillquit and Meyer London whom people in our row of hard benches murmured would "go far" in politics.

So the education of a young Brooklynite moved from a polyglot neighborhood and school to history-studded Prospect Park, the Brooklyn Museum of Arts and Science, the public library, the victrola with its treasures by Caruso, John McCormick, and Geraldine Farrar, the Metropolitan Opera House, Keith's vaudeville theatre, and glamorous old Gotham.

Just before the vistas of high school opened, I was sitting on the tennis lawn on a free-floating Saturday afternoon. Someone dropped a newspaper on the grass. It was August 5, 1914, and the huge type of the *New York American* screamed: ENGLAND DECLARES WAR ON GERMANY. The few who read it muttered something about those crazy Germans and the crazier Kaiser. Someone in England wrote of that day: "The lights went out all over the world." But in Brooklyn it was a brave, bright, sunny August day.

WALTER BROMBERG: LIFE EVENTS

1900	Born December 16 in New York City
1925	B.S., University of Cincinnati
1926	M.D., Long Island Medical College (now Down-state Medical Center, State University of New York)
1926-1928	Medical and surgical internship; resident neurologist, Mount Sinai Hospital, New York
1928-1930	Junior physician, Manhattan State Hospital, New York
1930-1942	Junior, then senior psychiatrist, Bellevue Psychiatric Hospital, New York
1930-1935	Clinical assistant, Vanderbilt Clinic, Columbia University
1933-1942	Instructor and assistant professor of clinical psychiatry, New York University College of Medicine
1933-1942	Director of Psychiatric Clinic of the Court of General Sessions, New York
1936-1942	Private practice, neuropsychiatry, New York
1937	Consultant to U.S. Bureau of Narcotics, Washington Diplomate, American Board of Psychiatry and Neurology. Published *The Mind of Man*
1937-1941	Analysand and candidate, New York Psychoanalytic Institute
1939	Published *Mind Explorers*
1942-1946	U.S. Armed Forces induction station, San Fran-

	cisco; U.S. Naval Reserve lieutenant commander and commander (Medical Corps active duty)
1945-1951	Group for Advancement of Psychiatry, member of Forensic Psychiatry Committee
1946-1950	Private practice, neuropsychiatry, Reno, Nevada
1948	Published *Crime and the Mind*
1950-1951	Clinical director, Mendocino State Hospital, Talmadge, California
1952-present	Private practice, psychiatry, psychotherapy, medical-legal consultant, Sacramento, California
1953-1961	B'nai Brith, past president, David Lubin chapter
1962	Life fellow of American Psychiatric Association. Published *The Nature of Psychotherapy*
1966-1969	Associate professor of psychiatry, Downstate Medical Center, State University of New York. Psychiatrist in charge, Prison Ward, Kings County Hospital, Brooklyn, New York
1968	Published *Psychiatric Aspects of Criminality*
1971-present	Adjunct professor of legal medicine, McGeorge School of Law, University of the Pacific
1973	American Academy of Psychiatry and Law Golden Apple award for distinguished contributions to psychiatry and law
1978-present	Member and vice president, the board of directors, American Board of Forensic Psychiatry
1979	Published *The Uses of Psychiatry in the Law*
1981	American Psychiatric Association Guttmacher Award

PSYCHIATRY BETWEEN
THE WARS, 1918-1945

1

EARLY DAYS

Psychiatry, like other branches of medicine, seems to have advanced in spectacular spurts that have followed long periods of stagnation. Traditional methods continue their unrewarding efforts until sudden flashes of inspiration open up vistas that illuminate old problems and provide fresh insights. Such a situation occurred in the 1790s, when William Tuke, a Quaker tea-merchant, decided to combat the bleeding-restraint routine then practiced and opened the York Retreat in England, thus initiating a regimen of encouragement, kindliness, and management by "moral means."[1] Another such period followed the unfolding of clinical neurology in the 1870s, when Jean Martin Charcot studied the lame and the halt in the Salpêtrière in Paris; still another occurred with Emil Kraepelin's unification of clinical psychiatry during the 1890s.

The history of psychiatry and medicine is dotted with events that have generated excitement and enthusiasm and have stimulated new trends and new viewpoints. One of these cycles followed World War I and lasted until World War II. This cycle saw the veritable burgeoning of psychiatry. This is the story of that epoch, during which alienism and psychiatry were lifted from a netherland of asylum practice and fumbling therapeutics to a high plateau of acute insights and startling methods of treatment.

For the first two decades of this century, the psychiatric scene, with a few exceptions to be discussed presently, could be best described as chaotic. Practicing psychiatrists were practically non-existent, except in state hospitals and private asylums (sanataria); neurologists treated nervous patients with tonics and opium derivatives that alternated with hypnosis, suggestive therapy, and persuasion borrowed from French neurologists; medical men handled depressions and neuroses symptomatically. Alienists functioned in criminal trials, preferably celebrated ones, while the bulk of offenders passed through the criminal system without thought of mental study. Medical students considered mental problems to be beyond their ken, although thoughtful state hospital physicians were revising their disparate diagnoses to fit the precise Kraepelinian outline. The subject of insanity (in some quarters it was called the study of "lunacy") lay remote and mysterious on the far periphery of medicine.

Academic psychology, already separated from its parent philosophy, had begun to display a vivid interest in the functioning mind, in measuring intelligence, and in studying memory, personality aberrations, and behavior. G. Stanley Hall, under the Darwinian stimulus, delevoped genetic psychology in terms of the evolution of man's feelings and emotions, in contrast to more structural descriptions of mind. In his exhaustive work, *Adolescence,* which appeared in 1905, Hall described the mind as a growing thing, responding to physiological, societal, and educational pressures.[2] William McDougall described the instincts;[3] John Watson developed behaviorism,[4] thus denying the fixity of instincts; and James Cattell, Robert Yerkes, Edward Thorndike, and others experimented with the living mind in its various functions.[5] The vitality that William James brought to psychology and the discovery of multiple personalities by Morton Prince in his famous Sally Beauchamp case stimulated a decade of argument and rebuttal about the existence of a "coconscious," a concept related to the "subconscious."[6] Controversies in American academe, as well as among psychotherapists allied to scientific psychology, filled the *Journal of Abnormal Psychology* until the turn of the century, when Sigmund Freud's "unconscious" confronted James Jackson Putnam, Boris Sidis, and others of the Boston group. By 1911 the American Psychopathological Association had been formed under the leadership of Morton Prince. At their meetings leading neurologists and psychologists discussed the new discoveries of a subliminal mind in relation to mental abnormalities. The slender lead psychologists maintained in the study of these mysterious conditions passed to medical men as they diffidently and reluctantly turned their attention to "mind cure" and to the patients who sought it.[7] But the force that catapulted the need for, and the growth of, a new psychiatry came chiefly from World War I with its military tragedies, social dislocations, and psychological pressures.

PSYCHIATRY AND THE GREAT WAR

The Great War with its attendent horrors of trench warfare, poisoned gas, and Big Berthas reacted on men's minds as no other war in history. The enormity of the problem of mental reactions in soldiers dawned only slowly on the American command in Europe. By 1918 General Jack Pershing, chief of the American Expeditionary Forces, sent an urgent message back to the War Department: "Prevalence of mental disorders in replacement troops . . . suggest urgent importance of eliminating the unfit."[8] In Washington, D.C., Surgeon General M. W. Ireland had already commissioned Thomas Salmon, Pearce Bailey, and Stewart Paton to create a plan for the reduction of mental casualties. After studying British psychiatric war neuroses in 1917, Salmon stated: "The present war is the first in which the functional nervous diseases ("shell shock") have constituted a major medico-military problem."[9] Edward Strecker, later head of the psychiatric department of the University of Pennsylvania, described the task and the solution devised by the small cadre of neuropsychiatrists who were sent to France. At the beginning, Strecker wrote, "We had to pay dearly for our myopia" in not training more men in neurology and psychiatry. This defect was remedied by the development of short courses for newly commissioned medical officers. Weeding out the potentially unfit in the induction station was their first task. Overseas, the "sorting out of neuropsychiatric casualties" from the trenches became a prime consideration, and with it came the demand to return as many to the front lines as possible. Using simple methods, "persuasion, rest, hot food," an appeal to patriotism, and firm paternalism produced results.[10] "Extended individual attention," noted Strecker, was not possible on the battle field. Serious cases were removed to evacuation hospitals and thence to hospitals in the United States. "We dealt," wrote

Strecker, "with epileptics, dementia praecox, tabetics, psychoneurotics, imbeciles . . . even a general who developed a manic state."[11]

In retrospect, Thomas Salmon, chief psychiatrist in the medical corps of the American Expeditionary Forces in France, wrote "[the] extraordinary effects of modern war upon the human nervous system . . . [are] responsible for not less than 20% of all discharges for disability."[12] In France he had encountered "guards armed with rifles and fixed bayonets in an observation ward, but. . . the clinical supervision of all mental cases has [now] been placed in our hands."[13] Wards once marked "Isolation Insane" were relabelled "Psychiatric Ward." Sidney Schwab after his return commented, "It is hoped that the fruits of the war experience in neuro-psychiatry may be translated, unweakened, and vitally intensified, into all civilian phases."[14]

The medical world was not prepared for the extensive emotional casualties of the war. Several European countries published reports by physicians at the front between 1915 and 1918 that commented on shock reactions, malingering, insanities, and the peculiar conditions of "unconsciousness and agitation with staring eyes . . . eventually diagnosed as hysterical."[15] In a Berlin letter to the *Journal of the American Medical Association,* dated April 1916 and entitled "Psychic Disturbance Incident to the War," a correspondent wrote that "a neutral Dutch psychiatrist reported 750,000 German soldiers and 1,600,000 civilians have been driven insane."[16] Although the numbers are probably apocryphal, all observers agreed that the enormous stress of shelling and trench warfare on the Western Front had taken its toll in nervous troubles. Pearce Bailey, an eminent neurologist, then a major in the United States Expeditionary Forces, reported in a 1917 *Harper's Magazine* that American psychiatric casualties were not "due to interference with nerves but in the willing, i.e., the neurasthenia and hysteria" of men in the trenches and under fire of German artillery.[17] The Great War focused attention on mental abnormalities short of insanity and hastened the effectiveness of the mental hygiene movement, which until then had dallied on a reform level supported by a handful of dedicated professionals and visionary citizens. It is not too much to say that the mental hygiene movement did not become a meaningful social movement until "shell shock" was recognized as a serious issue among returning soldiers.

Prior to the war, the National Committee for Mental Hygiene had started collecting information about mental patients in the various states. The stimulus came in part from Clifford Beers's book, *A Mind That Found Itself,* which exposed the "existing evils in the care of the mentally ill."[18] In 1917 Dr. Salmon, investigating a county poor farm in a southern state as a part of his duties for the national committee, found "a yard man, formerly a trolley car conductor, taking care of the insane . . . three or four remained in cages all day, on stone floors instead of on green grass."[19] While the fate of mental defectives and the "unfortunate" insane in state institutions attracted attention and stirred some sympathy, the number of young men suffering nervous disabilities in veteran's hospitals brought the message home.

By 1918 the propaganda campaign had already begun. The attitude that mental illness was no more blameworthy than the measles was promulgated by pamphlets, lectures, the child guidance movement, and the official journal of the mental hygiene movement, *Mental Hygiene.* Professor William James had already extolled the movement in consonance with his "healthy-mindedness" approach to mental vacillations and doubts. Adolf Meyer, who first suggested the name "mental hygiene" for the movement, became an active supporter, as did a few leading psychiatrists.

William James's philosophic pragmatism fitted the tenor of the mental health message. His teachings reflected an optimism that ran like a leitmotif through the efforts of mental hygienists. "Let us make our nervous system our ally instead of our enemy," James wrote. He argued for an "attitude of utility," a way of thinking that *worked.*[20] Although he spoke to teachers, he also talked to America. Indeed, a certain degree of "bullishness," even euphoria, pervaded the mental hygiene movement of the period.

Returning from the war, Dr. Salmon poured his energies into the movement. As his biographer E. D. Bond wrote, "Psychiatry was to be the leader in the emancipation of the mentally stricken." Salmon himself wrote, "It has an important part to play in the great movements for social betterment . . . for the feebleminded, eugenics, inebriety, management of abnormal children . . . leadership in the problems of treatment of criminals, prevention of crime, prostitution, dependency."[21]

Mental hygiene was raised to the level of reform, as it touched tangentially on several social programs brought to the public's attention.

INFLUENCE OF REFORM MOVEMENTS

The fervor with which psychiatric protagonists attacked brutality and neglect of the insane spread across the country. Social reform was in the air from eugenics to education, from suffrage for women to prohibition. Prison reform, closely allied to psychiatry, concerned many. Thomas Mott Osborne, the warden of Sing Sing State Prison, made a sincere effort to humanize prisons in the New York system after he spent one week as a voluntary inmate in Auburn State Prison. Placed in an isolation cell after a minor infraction, he encountered "a dark cell [with] no seat, no bed, no mattresses, no water, a hard floor, and a bucket. . . . we were given three gills of water for 24 hours (before 1913 the convicts were given one gill for 24 hours) and one piece of bread."[22] When released, he experienced an "overwhelming sense of the hideous cruelty of the whole barbaric, brutal business." Spearheading the prison reform movement, Osborne earned enemies, but he also made progress. He recognized the mental nature of the problem: "Courts make serious mistakes when psychological elements of the case are not taken into consideration."[23]

While the clergy echoed Osborne's plea for more light on the "darker side of human affairs,"[24] Dr. Bernard Glueck at the Government Hospital for the Insane in Washington, D.C., and later at Sing Sing Prison in New York studied the mental disorders of prisoners "under stressful conditions." His work in Washington led him to question "whether the habitual criminal does not belong rather in a hospital than a prison."[25] His analysis of 608 prisoners in Sing Sing Prison in which he detailed their personality profiles, was a landmark in psychiatric criminology, an unheard of field in 1918.[26]

Other reforms, such as Prohibition, found approbation among the public. An editorial comment in a 1920 *Literary Digest* exulted,

"The precise effect of the passing of John Barleycorn . . . has brought the manifold blessings of increased bank-savings in the place of barroom wastage."[27]

The problem of alcoholism, inebriety, or drunkenness, as it was commonly called at the time, had worried psychiatrists as a basic problem in mental disease for many years. In 1911 William A. White wrote, "Alcohol and syphilis taken together are generally regarded as being responsible for twenty-five per cent of the insane."[28] For this reason Prohibition was regarded as a public good. Even more highly regarded for the prevention of insanity was sterilization to rid the generations of so-called unfit persons. Riding on the fervor of eugenics, mental defectives, epileptics, and the morally degenerate, "habitual criminals," could be involuntarily sterilized in sixteen states by 1917.[29] In an oft quoted case in Virginia wherein sterilization was ordered for inmates in mental institutions, Justice Oliver Wendell Holmes of the United States Supreme Court stated: "It is better for the world, if, instead of waiting to execute degenerate offspring . . . society can prevent those who are manifestly unfit from continuing their kind."[30]

One area of reform, preventive medicine, had not yet invaded public consciousness. The discovery of vitamins by Casimir Funk in 1913, their role in deficiency diseases, and after much experimentation the insistence of Joseph Goldberger and his associates on the importance of a proper diet in 1920, remained outside the ken of practicing physicians.[31] There were predecessors to these scientists: Weir Mitchell had clamored years earlier for "good food" for neurasthenics, which he prescribed in his rest cure. Inveighing against the "frying pan . . . which reigns supreme west of the Alleghenies," he spoke against hasty and ill-cooked foods.[32]

In the mid-nineteenth century the notion of "venereal excess" and its deleterious effect on all the organs of the body, which, it was believed, produced "languor, lassitude, muscular relaxation, general debility . . . hypochondria . . . feebleness of all the senses" was widespread. Sylvester Graham of Graham bread fame joined vegetarianism with proscriptions against "amative excesses . . . even at a proper age . . . between married couples" because it might result in "exhaustion of the nervous powers."[33] But there were only a few mavericks in the medical profession in the early twentieth century who harped on the dangers of adulterated foods. Elmer Lee and Charles A. Tyrell published a lay magazine called *Health* around 1903, in which they espoused the cause of brown sugar, brown rice, and fruit juices to combat "refined foods."[34] Drs. Lee and Tyrell found the dire consequences of a "wrong diet" even reached into psychiatric fields: "Wrong diet . . . is the chief cause of abnormal sexuality. . . . Too stimulating foods excite the nerves . . . sex pleasures and immorality result from stimulation. . . . Stimulation is inflammation. . . . Unnatural foods heat the blood. . . ." In 1906 the Pure Food and Drug Act was enacted by Congress after years of struggles with vested interests. In this endeavor Harvey Wiley took the lead.

Most significant for those in the forefront of the hygienic reform movement was the ubiquitous abuse of patent medicines for emotional disquiet, failing sexual powers, depression, and any human ill. The hold that proprietary medicines exerted on the American public, even as late as the second decade of this century, is difficult to exaggerate. In 1917 the American Medical Association was moved to expose the most blatant of such nostrums on the basis of their alcoholic and opium derivative content and therapeutic uselessness. In a report headed "Propaganda for Reform," a pharmacological committee of the AMA reported that Pain's Celery Compound, advertised as the "True Nerve Tonic, for disease arising from a debilitated nervous system," contained 16 to 20 percent alcohol and that Dr. Craig's Nerve Pills for "Brain Fag . . . nervous prostration" contained a similar amount of alcohol.[35]

PUBLIC ATTITUDES TOWARD MENTAL ILLNESS

Yet this renewed emphasis on removing man's social-psychic blemishes was not evident in the daily life of the average American during the early 1920s. More particularly, reform influences, although clearly perceptible in retrospect, had little direct relation to neuropsychiatry as a clinical field. The average citizen with no personal contact with mental disease had little concern with the rising tide of interest in psychology. The man in the street and the woman in the home experienced measles, scarlet fever, pneumonia, and blood poisoning, but their knowledge of psycho-pathology as such was limited to gothic tales of insane asylums or passed off as eccentricities. The problems of the insane, the psychopathic, or the mentally impaired were not unrecognized, but they remained hidden from view just as the insane themselves were locked behind gray walls. Caretakers of the insane were doctors who, it was assumed, could not practice medicine outside asylum walls. If insanity occurred in one's family, it was submerged as a dark secret or excused in a young person as the second term of the genius = insanity equation that Max Nordau, a Hungarian psychiatrist, had proclaimed in the 1890s to be the end product of human degeneracy.[35]

Nordau's popularization of the degeneracy theory was built on the pioneer work of Augustin Morel, a French psychiatrist who in 1860 established hereditary weaknesses passed on from generation to generation as the cause of insanity. He identified certain stigmata as evidence of degeneracy: subnormal bodily build, deformed skull, badly formed ears (the Morel ear) and palate, irregular teeth, "snake-like eyes," even an abnormally long appendix. The degeneration theory pervaded psychiatry during the last half of the nineteenth century and provided an "element of fatalism," as Gregory Zilboorg put it.[37] Cesare Lombroso reinforced the concept by describing the stigmata characteristic of the so-called born criminal, the atavistic man, by adding "ferocious looks, thin upper lip, crooked nose, voluminous jaw, low brow."[38] Although Eugen Bleuler in the early twentieth century decried these indices of degeneracy in writing that they "merged into false paths," they had a sinister effect on the public's feelings toward mental abnormalities.[39] The triad of horrors associated with Lombroso's writings—atavism, depravity, and moral imbecility, which was associated with alcoholism and poverty—struck deeply in the preconscious of the public.

At the same time other notions were abroad about mental and physical infirmities. Neurasthenia and hysteria, as diagnoses of nervous afflictions, had gained currency among the public who understood neurasthenia to mean a kind of cowardly weakness and hysteria to be a condition any female could assume for reasons adequate to herself. In general, the notion of mental illness as the offshoot of depravity somewhere in the family tree continued to prevail. An editorial writer in *California and Western Medicine* commented in 1924 on the "old-fashioned view that insanity inflicted a terrible disgrace upon the individual and family and implied a taint that was transmitted and could hardly be eradicated."[40]

Lesser degrees of nervous troubles were handled by general practitioners; kindly family doctors examined, counselled, reassured, and medicated with bromides, luminal, or whatever produced symptomatic relief, or recommended a change of scene—a sea voyage for those who could afford it, the mountains or the seashore for others. The multitude of gastrointestinal and genitourinary symptoms, expressed as biliousness, sick headache, dyspepsia, spermatorrhea, nervous exhaustion, depression, neuralgia, spasms, and nerve weakness, were treated with tonics and sedatives or nostrums of uncertain content by patent medicine vendors. Some family doctors were less solicitous. Our family practitioner, a stern man educated in Germany and therefore completely scientific, choked off any descriptive reports of feelings or emotional failings by shoving a tongue depressor into his patients' mouths. With his Prussian crew cut and no-nonsense manner, he disposed of nervous complaints with a gruff "hummph." While he took the pulse, pulled down a lower eyelid to examine for anemia, his heavily browed eyes glared his patient into silence.

In the main, psychotherapy early in the century belonged to nonmedical persons, religious and educational leaders who utilized an inspirational format. The Emmanuel movement, Unity, Theosophy, Mental Science, Christian Science, and the New Thought movement, which, spurred by reports of successes with hypnosis and suggestive therapy, rested its case on influencing the "subconscious" to overcome doubts and nervous symptoms, captured the imagination of many. Professor James too recognized the value of mind cure: "The plain fact remains that the spread of the movement has been due to the practical fruits, and the extremely practical turn of character of the American People," although he went on to caution that a "good deal of mind-cure literature . . . is so moon-struck with optimism . . . that an academically trained intellect finds it almost impossible to read."[41] He confessed, however, that he tried "eighteen sittings" with mind cure for his recurrent depressions.

Most mind-cure systems relied on direct acceptance of help from the Deity, some on the recently discovered "subconscious," and others, like the one developed by John Rathbone, an Episcopal minister, physician, and psychiatrist, applied faith and suggestion to emotionally distraught patient-petitioners.[42] Curiously, the development of pastoral psychiatry stirred complaints among some of the clergy. Religious educators, realizing that those teachings to youth concerning "character building" had to proceed on a moral and psychological basis, objected to the intrusion of psychiatry, or at least psychiatrically trained men, into their field. James West, a youth leader writing on the church, the child, and motion pictures states, "The big need [in motion pictures] is that right conduct be emotionalized. . . . [We need] stories in which self-sacrifice becomes glorious, truthfulness and honesty commendable . . . fairness honorable . . . [and] the lack of it despicable."[43] Not only religious leaders and educators but also politicians, like President Hoover, urged the youth of America to have "confidence in right-mindedness."[44]

Surreptitiously, religious leaders borrowed the mental hygiene notion of "right thinking" for use in their counseling; educators swallowed the idea whole. I can remember the persistent efforts of my primary grade teacher to instill moral values in us by repeating frequently, "Reputation is what the world thinks of you; character is what God knows of you!" James Beebe, a clergyman and a professor of Methodist theology, when lecturing on home visits to parishioners, enjoined his ministerial students to "be a good listener . . . to help discharge the load of pent-up emotion, loosen tension, and release strain, so the weary soul feels better."[45] There was more than a hint of the therapeutic attitude in such moral exhortations.

The intrusion of psychiatric thinking into moral training stimulated an awareness of the loosening grip that religious precepts exerted. In 1930 Thomas Beer complained in an article in *Scribner's Magazine* titled "Toward Sunrise" that "the cultivated classes . . . had abandoned Christianity. . . . As it now stands Christianity is moribund. . . . American society struggles toward a sunrise of mental comfort."[46] Pastoral psychiatrists echoed the complaint. Father Oliver in his *Pastoral Psychiatry and Mental Health* wrote, "[whereas] the daily presence of a priest in old Trinity Church in New York . . . to listen to anyone who cares to ask for any kind of help . . . [now] people hurry off to the office of the newest psychoanalyst. . . . it could not have happened twenty years ago."[47] A parish priest and clinician, he added thoughtfully, "Both have the essential quality of caring." In a more troubled vein, James Preston asked in an article fortuitously titled "D.D. versus M.D.," why "the twentieth century mind believes more and more in psychotherapy than in God. There are many young men and women . . . who are taking their difficulties by the scruff of the neck and are turning away from the church because it no longer seems to help them face the realities of living."[48]

There was cause for complaint among churchmen. The tide of humanism threatened to sweep psychology and psychotherapy into its bosom. Walter Lippmann in his *Preface to Morals* placed the new attitude in clear perspective: "The humanistic view rests on human psychology and an interpretation of human experience . . . detachment, understanding. . . . a disinterested mind is harmonious with itself and reality" as opposed to what he described as "theocratic culture."[49] Psychiatry itself was not particularly involved in this controversy of religion versus psychology, but the slow loosening of traditional religious attitudes undoubtedly aided the acceptance of a psychological view of man during these decades.

So the move for self-understanding via mind healing rolled on, combining oriental mysticism with plagiarized bits of psychology and psychoanalysis. Lee Steiner reviewed the extent of irregular practitioners of the healing arts in 1940 and estimated that 15 to 20 million Americans were influenced by theosophy and other mystic-spiritualistic therapeutic methods.[50] To judge by Mark Twain's caustic comment at the turn of the century that "it is a reasonably safe guess that in America in 1920 there will be 10 million Christian Scientists . . . trebled in 1930 . . .[to] be politically formidable in 1940—to remain that permanently," religio-spiritualistic healing methods were equally widespread during the 1900s.[51] Sincere efforts to use the powers of religious belief to remove depression and other so-called nervous symptoms were extended by "applied psychologists" who ventured into areas of personality development with claims of conferring "health, vibrancy, and business success" on their adherents. Books like F. C. Haddock's *Power of the Mind* swung away from faith healing into a therapy aimed at eliminating their client's "inferiority complex."

Less blatant and more soundly based was Émile Coué's auto-suggestion. Coué, trained at the Nancy clinic of Dr. Ambrose-Auguste Liébault, was regarded by an English follower in 1922 as using a "scientific discovery based on psychology . . . not a pseudo-religion like Christian Science or 'New Thought'."[52] His formula, "Every day in every way, I feel better and better," was repeated rapidly over and over as a whirring sound exerted a hypnotic effect. His rooms in Nancy were crowded by American and European visitors. One Mrs. Kirk left a report of her obser-vations of Coué's technique: " 'You have been sowing bad seeds in your Unconscious, now you will sow good seed,' he would say calmly."[53] She prophesied, "Monsieur Coué will find a hearty welcome next month in America," but she also noted that the *Journal of the American Psychiatric Association* called his method "cloudy stuff." When this modest man came to America, his success was enormous—and transient.

Medical practitioners were not unmindful of such developments. The *Journal of the American Medical Association* carried an article by Dr. William House in 1920 complaining that the "world suffers from disarticulations resulting from World War. . . . The rising tide of occultism, mysticism, ouija board, metaphysics, telepathy, miracle healing . . . are used for troublesome symp-toms."[54] More pointedly, the doctor commented: "Clairvoyance and spiritualism are a refuge for incipient insanity among the senile and middle aged." In the same year, an editorial writer in the journal cynically assailed the "newer quackery [that provides] health and happiness through commercialized psychology . . . women suffering from ennui of idleness, faces elaborated with artifices . . . to stimulate the lost buoyancy of youth." The editorial went on to warn: "People are paying too much attention nowadays to the MIND. . . . Fascination for cognition on things sexual [contains] elements of danger."[55]

Outstanding neurologists also took note of the "new quackery." Frederick Peterson, early a friend of psychoanalysis, included the latter in a 1919 article entitled "Credulity and Cures," in which he took physicians to task for accepting such cures as the "tar water cure" or excision of the ovaries for psychoneurotic troubles.[56] His indignation over doctors who removed nasal turbinates or performed clitoridectomies for "nervous disorders" or trephined the skull of mental defectives "under the impression the brain would grow if given more room" was no less than it was for psychoanalysis. This method, he opined, would "take its place in our historical medical museum along with the other curiosities which the centuries have accumulated." His article, which was featured in the *Journal of the American Medical Association,* criticized physicians for their lack of "critical faculty" more than the patient-public in its beliefs and wishes for magical cures.

PSYCHIATRY AND THE LITERATI

While American medical officialdom was protecting gullible physicians from the "new psychology" (Dr. Kellogg of Battle Creek, Michigan, had declared earlier that sexual activity for a man of fifty invited early senescence), the literate public's relation to psychiatry and psychology was more friendly. The writings of William James were known to educated persons as an amalgam of philosophy and psychology, as was the Terman revision of the Binet-Simon Intelligence Test and the army's Alpha Test that popularized the designation "moron." Thus informed, many could appreciate H. L. Mencken's chortling over the American "boo-boisie" and his delight in cynically describing the mental level of the vast American hinterland as moronic. This same public also knew something of erotica through Havelock Ellis's *Psychology of Sex* and Richard Krafft-Ebing's work on perversions, shrouded though it was in Latinisms. Special editions of pornographia were held privately by collectors.

Public and college libraries locked these and less candid books behind closed bookcases, but the more adventurous of the reading public managed to read Radclyffe Hall's *The Well of Loneliness,* slake their curiosity on Henry Miller's *Tropic of Cancer*, and peer into the unexpurgated edition of Frank Harris's *The Story of My Love Life.* Harris's coy account of his sexual conquests and Miller's liberal use of four-letter words qualifed their works (both

published in Paris) as "dirty books" with a limited circulation.
Those books "limited strictly to members of recognized professions," such as W. F. Robie's *The Art of Love*, were essentially
educational. Robie's volume explained the Karma method of sexual intercourse (India), the Karezza technique of *coitus reservatus,*
and included confessions of his own uninhibited sexual activities.[57]
Although such works were not directly related to psychoanalytic
theory, this type of erotic literature was imputed to Sigmund
Freud's influence.

In view of this attitude, it is understandable that the avant-
garde were attracted to psychoanalysis more than to more mundane
aspects of clinical psychiatry; they were, however, equally balanced
by the detractors. Richard Le Gallienne, writing in *Harper's
Magazine* in 1921, fastidiously pointed out that "legal and physiological terms as 'reaction' should be left in vocabularies from
which [they] have been dug out."[58] His dislike of the "hideous
word 'inhibition' . . . the screech of which is everywhere" was
matched by his loathing of "Freud with his 'complexes' . . . and
various other nastinesses . . . 'motivation' too is a horrible word."
But this plaint was not unusual in a period that Samuel Eliot
Morison has called the "Great Change" in America, when sexual
and social mores changed dramatically, religious sanctions
weakened, and the prevailing "Protestant ethos . . . was crumbling
from within."[59]

In New York City the epicenter for Morison's "Great Change"
was located in Greenwich Village. A haven for poets, writers,
philosophic anarchists, and fellow travelers who embraced the
new spirit of freedom, Greenwich Village promised relief from
social inhibitions. Eccentricity was tolerated, even admired, as in
the case of Maxwell Bodenheim whose novel, *Replenishing Jessica,*
had been rescued from a legal charge of "indecent writing." The
attraction of Greenwich Village was obviously prurient on the part
of the "uptown" public. Artists and writers found the atmosphere
congenial to their production of serious work, but the public was
titillated by the fantasy of implied sexual freedom. As Albert
Parry in his comprehensive *Garrets and Pretenders, A History of
Bohemianism in America* wrote, "the public gulped . . . the facts
of sin . . . with a vicarious thrill because they wanted to be like
those free-loving Villagers but dared not."[60]

The magnet that drew New York's youthful intellectual aspirants to the Village passed beyond the promise of sexual freedom. It led to freedoms in art, literature, the theater, life-style and conversation, disguised though they were on occasion. I remember attending a poetry reading by Maxwell Bodenheim in the flat of one of his admirers. Bodenheim, his conjunctiva slightly inflamed by bad "booze," read with the air of a seer, while we listened, glad to be on the cutting edge of literary progress. On the other hand, artists of the rank of Ben Shahn, scholars like Albert Parry (who later became professor of Russian at Colgate University), novelists Dawn Powell, Clement Wood, and others whom I met were genuinely interested in the new literary forms, psychoanalysis, and the American social-political scene.

Novelists had, of course, always dealt with the morbid in their American prototypes. Edgar Lee Masters in his 1915 *Spoon River Anthology* and Sherwood Anderson in his 1921 *Triumph of the Egg* described the hidden perversions and eccentricities (read "psychopathology") of their characters in small-town America. Many authors in the 1920s and 1930s wrote novels on the wings of "Freudian inspiration," which to Bernard De Voto, Harvard literary critic, represented merely "one of the fads that periodically rage through the antechambers and subbasements of literature."[61] Although authors of this vintage "had an honorable part in the struggle to liberate American literature from the pruderies that hampered it," De Voto noted, only James Joyce in *Ulysses* plumbed the "workings of the mind . . . through interactions of various levels of consciousness." But pruderies prevented *Ulysses* from being published in the United States until 1933 (*U.S. v. Ulysses, Random House, Inc.*), when Judge John M. Woolsey of the U.S. District Court for the Southern District of New York ruled against its suppression. The government had considered the book obscene because of its Anglo-Saxon terms. Judge Woolsey in an elegant and perceptive decision ruled in favor of recognizing the importance of the subconscious in human affairs:

Joyce has attempted—it seems to me, with astonishing success—to show how the screen of consciousness with its ever-shifting kaleidoscopic impressions carries, as it were on a plastic palimpsest, not only what is in focus of each man's observation of the actual things about him, but also a penumbral zone residua of past impressions, some recent and some drawn up by association from the domain of the subconscious.

It is my considered opinion . . . whilst in many places the effect of Ulysses on the reader undoubtedly is somewhat emetic, nowhere does it tend to be aphrodisiac.

Nevertheless, some writers were incensed at the adoption of this kind of psychologic free association. G. K. Chesterton, for example, in 1923 blasted "Freudian intellectual bullies . . . with their monomania of sex. . . .Psychoanalysis can no longer be dismissed as a fad; it has risen to the dignity of a fashion. It stands now in the open street, visible to the man in the street like some florid . . . tailor's dummy outside a tailor's shop. . . . It is time somebody knocked the stuffing out of it."[62] More soberly, Water Lippmann, writing in 1915, caught the pitch of the reading public's reaction: "This uncanny wisdom [of psychoanalysis] is to most people both fascinating and horrible. They can neither take hold nor let go."[63]

While the tides of opinion about the "new psychology" shifted back and forth among literateurs, especially in New York, a spirit of emancipation grew among the public. It is more than probable that the acceptance of psychiatry and psychoanalysis in America had much to do with the new freedom and changed life-style following World War I. Mark Sullivan neatly summarized the psychological ambience of the twenties when he wrote, "Psychology in the Twenties suffered a sea change. . . . Instead of preoccupation with the pathological, psychology began to take an interest in the average man, to explain what he was, to show him profitable ways of thinking and conducting himself."[64] Thus when Freud's Introductory Lectures reached American readers in A. A. Brill's 1916 translation, it produced a sense of liberation as if a veil had been lifted on an area muted by the suppression evident in the post-Victorian period. Nowhere had this suppression been more severe than among physicians purporting to treat sexual problems in the young. G. Stanley Hall in a footnote reported on a pamphlet distributed at the fifty-ninth annual session of the American

Medical Association in 1902 and "approved by eight well-known physicans who discussed it." According to the pamphlet:

> If a boy friend boasts to you of his sexual experience with girls, drop his acquaintance at once. . . . If a boy in an unguarded moment tries to entice you to masturbatic experiences, he insults you. Strike him at once, and beat him as long as you can stand. . . . Forgive him in your mind, but never speak to him again. . . . If a man scoundrel suggests indecent things, slug him with a stick or stone or anything else at hand. Give him a scar that all may see, and if you are arrested, tell the judge all, and he will approve your act, even if it is unlawful. . . . If a villain shows you a filthy book or picture, snatch it from him and give it to the first policeman you meet. . . . If a vile woman invites you . . . you cannot strike her, but think of a poisonous, glittering snake. . . . She is a degenerate and probably diseased, even a touch may poison you and your children.[65]

THE CONTINUED STRUGGLE

In spite of medical caution that approached exhortation, literary allusions to sexual liberation attracted the attention of the reading public. The writings of James Branch Cabell, particularly his *Jurgen,* were enjoyed by budding intellectuals because of their veiled symbolism: The lance of Jurgen became a phallic symbol. The suppression of *Jurgen* after its publication for its "free-and-easy sexual morality" coincided with the alarm that psychoanalysis was assumed to foster.[66] Reaction to Cabell's writings was almost as vivid as that to psychoanalysis. Carl Van Doren, a literary critic, wrote of *Jurgen*, "The rage of a few zealots has directed attention to certain phallic passages in the narrative . . . only the nimble-snouted root them out."[67] Still, popular books and articles in increasing numbers poured off the presses. Public taste in psychologic reading was whetted as the 1920s advanced. Not only did nonmedical persons promote knowledge of the subconscious and how it affected daily life, but competent physicians began to explain psychoanalysis to the literate public. Burt Farnsworth in a work titled *Practical Psychology for Men and Women in the Industries and Professions and for the General Reader* explained the subconscious as containing "knowledge and skill which we have acquired, and all those experiences of which we have been conscious but for the moment are not."[68] Andre Tridon, a physician with psychiatric experience, also wrote a popular book, *Psychoanalysis and Behavior*, in which he "interpreted human conduct from a psychoanalytic point of view."[69]

The spate of popularizations of psychoanalysis continued from the 1920s until well into the 1930s. For example, Louis Bisch, a psychiatrist with a degree in psychology as well, wrote *Your Inner Self* in 1922, which explained in simple terms such Freudian mechanisms as condensation, displacement, free association, *Lapsus linguae,* and so forth; and W. Beran Wolfe, who had ably translated several of Alfred Adler's works, published a volume in 1933 entitled *Nervous Breakdown: Its Cause and Cure*, dedicated to "Men and Women in Perplexity."[70] Writing from an Adlerian point of view with "plain words to patients," Dr. Wolfe sought to bring to his readers the benefits of psychotherapy. The tone of the book was sometimes hortatory, sometimes pleading, but essentially aimed at illuminating the nature of the all too common "nervous breakdown." Wolfe wrote: "Thousands of people are walking the streets at this minute, suffering from a nervous breakdown, too ignorant to know that something is wrong, or too stubborn, or too proud, to see an expert."[71] The cases Wolfe described, typical phobias, anxiety reactions, and hysterias, were related in a straight-forward manner with a paucity of technical terms that was intended to remove the mystery surrounding nervous afflictions. He and other popularizers spoke to people in their own language, reassuring them that the closely guarded authority of the physician in matters therapeutic could also yield to a feeling of humanness. It was a kind of unofficial mental hygiene that reached a wide audience.

Other medical writers, explaining the by now familiar neuroses, eschewed the psychoanalytic approach, basing their advice and reassurance on more commonplace attitudes. Dr. William Sadler, a Chicago surgeon turned psychiatrist in his later years, published a book in 1929, titled *The Mind at Mischief: Tricks and Deceptions of the Subconscious and How to Cope with Them*. He based his exposition on simple principles; in discussing the various clinical neuroses and their causes, he said, "I have no hesitancy in setting down the inheritance of an unstable nervous system . . . [and] the lack of proper training in the nursery" as the cause of these ubiquitous troubles.[72] As a dim reflection of the conflict going on within the medical fraternity over dynamic psychiatry, Sadler dedicated his book to "patients . . . to assist the layman in understanding . . . [and] to be helpful to men and women struggling with the intellectual vagaries and contending with 'complexes' causing them serious troubles." Even more doctrinaire was the tone in a book entitled *The Normal Child and How to Keep it Normal in Mind and Morals* by the prestigious neurologist, Dr. Bernard Sachs of New York. Dr. Sachs addressed his book to parents on behalf of children and attacked psychoanalytic theories as a substitute for wholesome, emotional relationships in a family-setting. In a chapter called "The Evils of Psychoanalysis," he wrote, "The Oedipus complex is a mere fabrication. . . . psychoanalysis is based on two false conceptions, infantile sexuality and the erotic dream."[73] While the more moderate Dr. J. F. Meagher, president of the Brooklyn Neurologic Society, in a letter to the *Journal of the American Medical Association* in 1921 said, "Criticism of the lay public's becoming too much interested in psychoanalysis is probably well taken, especially by lay magazine writers . . . [but] the battle raged about this subject is gradually coming into its own."[74]

One of the consequences of the upsurge of popularizations of psychoanalysis in the early 1920s was the number of untrained psychotherapists who interpreted their patients' dreams according to the book and undertook to liberate their repressions, which, in the words of Bernard Sachs, were "dragged into the limelight . . . to the delight of the practioner, but to the detriment of the young victim."[75] What came to be known as "wild analysis" was denounced by valid analysts and was the cause in part of Freud's gloomy comment that the "generally cordial reception accorded his theories in America was due to the absence of embedded scientific tradition."[76] Reading the works of Freud, Abraham, Jones, Ferenczi, and other accepted analysts, and applying them forthwith to patients so grew that psychoanalytic societies in New York, Boston, and elsewhere, actively repudiated "wild analysis."

Yet, without knowledge of the conflicts raging in medical academe, the reading public became at least superficially acquainted with analysis and therefore psychiatry. A fascination with new views of the human psyche spread from the East Coast to the larger cities in the Midwest and West. It became the mark of an educated citizenry, particularly in university circles, to be aware and even to take sides with the various schools of dynamic psychiatry. Neurologists, neuropsychiatrists, and clinical psychologists, struggled with choices afforded them. "We have many individual brands of [psychiatric] thinking" wrote a reviewer of Edward Kempf's book *Psychopathology*[77] in 1921, "Forel's hypnotism, Janet's dissociation, Sidis's hypnoidization, Prince's multiple personality, Freud's elaborate analytic system, Jung's analytic constructive vision, works on symbolism, etc., nosologists, like Kraepelin."[78]

But to the layman, the seeds of inquiry into the subterranean mind had been sown, and patients dissatisfied with older methods of psychotherapy—reassurance, tonics, sedatives, and placebos—created a need. By the end of the third decade of this century, "consumer sovereignty" (to borrow a phrase from John Kenneth Galbraith) seemed to have aided the burgeoning of psychiatry. Doctors experimented, theorized, and cogitated, while the public, eager to gain from psychiatric discoveries, asked in increasing numbers for admission to this psychic wonderland.

NOTES

1. See Samuel Tuke, *Description of the Retreat in the Institution in New York, for Insane Persons of the Society of Friends, Containing an Account of its Origin and Progress and Means of Treatment and Statement of Cases* (York, England, 1893).

2. Granville Stanley Hall, *Adolescence, its Psychology and its Relation to Physiology, Anthropology, Society, Sex, Religion and Education,* 2 vols. (New York: D. Appleton & Co., 1905).

3. William McDougall, *Outline of Psychology* (New York: Charles Scribner's Sons, 1923), p. 103.

4. John B. Watson, *Psychology from the Standpoint of a Behaviorist* (Philadelphia: J. B. Lippincott, 1919).

5. Gardner Murphy, *A Historical Introduction to Modern Psychology* (New York: Harcourt, Brace & Co., 1929).

6. Morton Prince, *The Dissociation of a Personality* (New York: Longmans, Green & Co., 1905).

7. Nathan G. Hale, Jr., *Freud and the Americans, The Beginning of Psychoanalysis in the United States, 1876-1917* (New York: Oxford University Press, 1971), chap. 9.

8. Nina Ridenour, *Mental Hygiene in the United States: A Fifty Year History* (Cambridge, Mass.: Harvard University Press, 1961).

9. Edward A. Strecker, "Military Psychiatry: World War I," in *One Hundred Years of American Psychiatry,* ed. J. K. Hall (New York: Columbia University Press, 1944), p. 385.

10. Ibid., p. 400.

11. Ibid., p. 404.

12. Thomas W. Salmon, "Some New Problems for Psychiatric Research in Delinquency," *Mental Hygiene* 4, no. 1 (January 1920): 29.

13. E. D. Bond, *Thomas Salmon, Psychiatrist* (New York: W. W. Norton, 1950), p. 104.

14. Sidney J. Schwab, "The Influence of War Upon Concepts of Mental Disease and Neurosis," *Mental Hygiene* 14, no. 8 (July 1920): 654.

15. Mabel W. Brown, *Neuro-Psychiatry and the War,* ed. Frankwood Williams (New York: National Com. Mental Hygiene, 1918).

16. Berlin Letter, "Psychic Disturbances Incident to the War," *Journal of the American Medical Association* (hereafter *JAMA*) 66 (April 29, 1916).

17. Pearce Bailey, "Psychiatry and the Army," *Harper's Magazine* 90 (July 1917): 251.

18. C. W. Beers, *A Mind That Found Itself,* 2d ed., (New York: Longmans, 1910).

19. Thomas W. Salmon, "A Country Poor Farm," *Mental Hygiene* 1, no. 1 (January 1917): 25.

20. William James, *The Energies of Man* (New York: Holt, 1916).

21. Bond, *Thomas Salmon, Psychiatrist,* p. 104.

22. Thomas M. Osborne, *Within Prison Walls* (New York: D. Appleton & Co., 1916), p. 245.

23. Thomas M. Osborne, *Society and Prisons* (New Haven: Yale University Press, 1916), p. 64.

24. *The Churchman,* quoted in *Literary Digest,* May 8, 1920, p. 52.

25. Bernard Glueck, *Studies in Forensic Psychiatry,* Criminal Science Monographs no. 2, American Institute of Criminal Law (Boston: Little, Brown & Co., 1916), p. 131.

26. Bernard Glueck, "A Study of 608 Admissions to Sing Sing Prison," *Mental Hygiene* 2 (January 1918): 85.

27. Editorial, *Literary Digest,* November 27, 1920, p. 38.

28. William A. White, "Preventive Principles in the Field of Mental Medicine," *Journal of the American Public Health Association* 1 (1911): 82.

29. Habitual Criminal Sterilization Act, *Laws of Oklahoma,* Title 57, Sec. 171 (1935).

30. Buck v. Bell, 274 U.S. 200 (1927).

31. Fielding Garrison, *History of Medicine,* 3d ed., rev. (Philadelphia: W. B. Saunders Co., 1921), p. 802.

32. Weir S. Mitchell, *Wear and Tear, or Hints for the Overworked* (Philadelphia: J. P. Lippincott, 1871).

33. Stephen Nissenbaun, *Sex, Diet and Debility in Jacksonian America* (Westport, Conn.: Greenwood Press, 1980), pp. 106, 162.

34. Elmer Lee and Charles A. Tyrell, *Health* (New York: Health Publications Co., 1903).

35. "Propaganda for Reform," *JAMA* 69 (November 10, 1917): 1636.

36. Max Simon Nordau, *Degeneration,* 4th ed., trans. of the 2d ed. (New York: D. Appleton & Co., 1895).

37. Gregory Zilboorg, *A History of Medical Psychology* (New York: W. W. Norton, 1941), p. 403.

38. Cesare Lombroso, *Crime: Its Causes and Remedies,* trans. H. P. Horton (Boston: Little, Brown & Co., 1911), p. 376.

39. Eugen Bleuler, *Textbook of Psychiatry*, trans. A. A. Brill (New York: Macmillan Co., 1924), p. 159.

40. Editorial, "The Treatment of Mental Diseases and Deficiencies," *California & Western Medicine* 12, no. 9 (September 1924): 462.

41. William James, *The Varieties of Religious Experience, A Study in Human Nature* (1902 reprint ed., New York: Modern Library, 1929), p. 94.

42. See John R. Oliver, *Pastoral Psychiatry and Mental Health* (New York: Charles Scribner's Sons, 1932), p. 298.

43. James E. West, "Character Building for the Youth of America," *The Motion Pictures* 1, no. 4 (January 1926): 1.

44. Herbert Hoover, Meeting, International Conference, reported in *The Motion Pictures* 1, no. 4 (January 1926): 4.

45. James A. Beebe, *The Pastoral Office* (New York: Methodist Book Concern, 1923), p. 159.

46. Thomas Beer, "Toward Sunrise, 1920-1930," *Scribner's Magazine* 87, no. 5 (May 1930): 536.

47. Oliver, *Pastoral Psychiatry,* p. 13.

48. James Preston, "D.D. vs. M.D.," *Scribner's Magazine* 87, no. 5 (May 1930): 554.

49. Walter Lippmann, *A Preface to Morals* (New York: Macmillan Co., 1929), p. 221.

50. Lee R. Steiner, *Where Do People Take Their Troubles* (New York: International University Press, 1945).

51. Mark Twain, *Christian Science* (New York: Harper & Bros., 1907), p. 72.

52. Harry C. Brooks, *The Practice of Autosuggestion by the Method of Émile Couré* (London: George Allen & Unwin, 1922), p. 4.

53. George E. Mowry, ed., *The Twenties: Fords, Flappers & Fanatics* (Englewood Cliffs, N.J.: Prentice-Hall, 1963), pp. 158-60.

54. William House, "Occultism and Insanity," *JAMA* 75, no. 2 (September 18, 1920): 127.

55. "Psychoanalysis," *JAMA* 76, no. 5 (January 29, 1921): 317.

56. Frederick Peterson, "Credulity and Cures," *JAMA* 73, no. 23 (December 6, 1919): 1737.

57. W. F. Robie, *The Art of Love,* (New York: Eugenia Press, 1921).

58. Richard Le Gallienne, "Words We Would Willingly Let Die," *Harper's Magazine* 143 (June 1921): 122.

59. Samuel Eliot Morison, *The Oxford History of the American People* (New York: Oxford University Press, 1965), p. 888.

60. Albert Parry, *Garrets and Pretenders, A History of Bohemia in America* (New York: Covici-Freide, 1933), pp. 312-14.

61. Bernard De Voto, "Freud in American Literature," *Psychoanalytic Quarterly* 9 (1940): 236-45.

62. Gilbert K. Chesterton, "The Game of Psychoanalysis," *Century Magazine* 106 (May 1923): 34-43.

63. Walter Lippmann, "Freud and the Layman," *New Republic* 2, suppl. 9 (April 17, 1915): 9.

64. Mark Sullivan, *Our Times,* vol. 6, *The Twenties* (New York: Charles Scribner's Sons, 1935), p. 424.

65. Hall, *Adolescence,* 1:470.

66. James B. Cabell, *Jurgen* (New York: McBride Co., 1919).

67. Carl Van Doren, *James Branch Cabell* (New York: McBride Co., 1925), p. 45.

68. Burt B. Farnsworth, *Practical Psychology for Men and Women in the Industries and for the General Reader* (New York: C. W. Clark, 1923).

69. Andre Tridon, *Psychoanalysis and Behavior* (New York: Alfred A. Knopf, 1921).

70. See Louis E. Bisch, *Your Inner Self* (New York: Page & Co., 1922), and Beran W. Wolfe, *Nervous Breakdown: Its Cause and Cure* (New York: Farrar & Rinehart, 1933).

71. Ibid., p. 171.

72. William S. Sadler, *The Mind at Mischief, Tricks and Deceptions of the Subconscious and How to Cope with Them* (New York: Funk and Wagnalls, 1929), p. 302.

73. Bernard Sachs, *The Normal Child and How to Keep it Normal in Mind and Morals* (New York: Paul Hoeber Co., 1926).

74. J. F. W. Meagher, "Letter," *JAMA* 76 no. 7 (February 12, 1921): 468.

75. B. Sachs, *The Normal Child,* p. 68.

76. Clarence P. Oberndorf, *A History of Psychoanalysis in America* (New York: Grune and Stratton, 1953), p. 130.

77. See Edward J. Kempf, *Psychopathology* (St. Louis: C. V. Mosby, 1920).

78. Book Review, *Archives of Neurology and Psychology* 5 (1921): 782.

2

THE NEUROLOGICAL HERITAGE

In spite of the public's newfound interest in psychotherapy and psychiatry, neither the study of nerve disease nor the
study of mental aberrations sprung into existence full-blown, like
Athena from the head of Zeus. For a century and more, both
fields had been tilled intensively but independently, until they came
together in a new clinical area called neuropsychiatry. Their
association was not without friction and contention. Because
neurologists had contributed a great deal to the field, and psychiatrists were relative newcomers, competition between the two
groups often was vigorous. Adolf Meyer, in retrospect, commented
on their mutual criticism when he wrote, "Some of the best [were]
hardly speaking to each other."[1] In 1894 Weir Mitchell, the dean
of American neurologists before the turn of the century, loosed
an attack on the complacency of asylum doctors at the annual
meeting of the American Medico-Psychological Association:
"Where, we ask, are your annual reports of scientific study, of
the psychology and pathology of your patients. . . . Seriously we
ask you experts, what have you taught us of the 91,000 insane
whom you see and treat?"[2] The answer by Walter Channing, a
spokesman for the asylum psychiatrists, was in kind: "[It is]
useless to expect neurologists will make successful executive officers
of insane hospitals. . . . It is not a question of knee-jerks or
ankle clonus or reaction time . . . but how to house the already
large numbers of insane."[3]

Three decades later the contentiousness still remained. Louis
Casamajor, one of New York's outstanding neurologists, recalled
that as psychiatry "boomed after World War I. . . . neurology . . .

shining in reflected glory . . . still refused to relax its grip on the private practice of psychiatry. The old mutual antagonism between the neurologist and the psychiatrist had not receded one inch."[4]

Writing from a neurologist's point of view, D. Denny-Brown, professor of neurology at Harvard Medical School, reported in retrospect a similar state of affairs: "The mounting aggressiveness of psychiatry soon encroached on what had been considered the neurologist's field, and by the 1930s . . . many predicted the extinction of the genus neurologists. . . . Many neurologists and neurologic departments became absorbed by departments of neurosurgery or else adopted the protective coloring in the form of the title "neuropsychiatrist" and still exist in unhappy dependence on these borderlands."[5]

The reasons for this dichotomy were philosophical, historical, and clinical. Neurologists could demonstrate their findings, measure or even weigh them in the autopsy room, but psychiatric observations could be described only in language that feebly reproduced the nuances of emotional life. Neurological theories were factual, based on neuropathology and neurophysiology: Psychiatric ideas and theories tended to be imaginative and transmitted in mythical, poetical, even novelistic language. The differences between the two groups were conceptual and methodological. Thus, Franz Nissl, a German neurologist, wrote in 1904, "As soon as we agree to see in all mental derangements the clinical expression of definite disease processes in the cortex, we remove the obstacles that make impossible agreement among alienists."[6] In contrast, a half-century later in 1954 Erwin Stengel, a psychoanalyst writing in the *British Journal of Psychology,* stated "Dynamic psychiatry is a psychiatry informed by psychoanalysis . . . in which psychological factors have largely taken the place previously held by heredity or hypothetical organic causes."[7] These opposing views—organic v. functional, and by extension neurology v. psychiatry—maintained their sharp edges through several decades of this century. Some, however, recognized a natural partnership. Dr. Langdon of Cincinnati in a 1903 report entitled "Neurological Progress and Prospects" that appeared in the *Journal of the American Medical Association* looked to "better facilities for teaching neurology, including psychology, psychiatry and psychotherapy" in medical schools.[8]

THE NEUROPSYCHIATRIC RAPPROCHEMENT

In spite of the conflict, many were convinced that abnormal conditions of mind and body could not be severed. In writing on syphilitic psychoses in 1916 Albert Barrett of the University of Michigan said, "Aside from structural influences of a syphilitic process in the nervous system . . . there is a possibility of psychogenic mental disturbance" in the individual confronting his infection.[9] The division of neurology from psychiatry receded in view of the complex symptoms of syphilis that involved both the body and the nervous system. Diagnoses of dementia paralytica (general paresis), locomotor ataxia (tabes dorsalis), and meningovascular lues and gumma, required psychiatric and neurological knowledge. Syphilis was known as the great imitator; every differential diagnosis of obscure medical conditions contained references to this protean disease. The *Archives of Neurology*, the *American Journal of Insanity* (changed in 1921 to *American Journal of Psychiatry*), and the *Journal of the American Medical Association* were filled with discussions of the diagnosis and treatment of syphilis of the central nervous system. Psychiatrists were called on to distinguish the extravagant delusions of the manic patient from those of the paretic. The slogan attributed to Osler, "know syphilis and you know medicine," was adopted by neurologists. B. P. Thom, a psychiatrist, wrote in 1921, "There is no psychosis that cannot be caused by syphilis," a concept that united both disciplines in this baffling field.[10]

The so-called neurasthenic syndrome, which included among its symptoms headache, dizziness, sleeplessness, irritability, lack of interest in work, and so forth, could and did occasionally represent the "prodromal signs of Paresis." Smith Ely Jelliffe and William A. White in their encyclopedic *Diseases of the Nervous System* wrote in indignation:

The neuropsychiater sees such patients who have had their teeth pulled, their tonsils gouged out, their eyes refitted, or eye muscles cut; their cervices amputated, their ovaries removed, from nine inches to six feet of gut cut out, all of the endocrine glands dispensed, orthopedic appliances applied, weeks of colonic irrigation, with or without electrical rigmaroles. Psychoanalyzed by the lay pretender, these patients often go through every fad and fiction of medicine before a competent examination reveals the underlying factor."[11]

All neurological textbooks, including the compendious book by Jelliffe and White, emphasized the clinical features of the various forms of central nervous system syphilis. In their fourth edition in 1923, they devoted ninety-two pages to the subject of lues and only twenty-one pages to tumors of the brain, which they called "relatively infrequent."[12] They appreciated, as did many other clinicians, that the discovery of the spirochete as the cause of paresis by Noguchi in 1911 clarified many obscure neurological conditions.[13] Still, they warned that the physician who concentrated on "amyotrophic lateral sclerosis, a failing memory, a persistent muscular atrophy of the arms, a protracted neuralgia, a failing eyesight, a progressive deafness, or a profound metabolic disorder, may readily overlook that syphilis is the unique cause for these syndromes."[14] Not everyone, however, agreed that the spirochete and general paralysis were related. William Malamud, reviewing this period, wrote: "Sporadic attempts to link up the disease and its bacteriological cause" were met by "almost fanatical resistance on the part of some of the eminent men of the time. The early ideas of the relation of general paralysis to alcoholism and a generally dissolute life persisted strongly."[15]

This issue of alcoholism and paresis was the subject of a study, entitled *Alcohol and Syphilis as Causes of Mental Disease* by George Kirby, in which he contrasted the incidence of mental disease between the 1910 and 1920 admissions to Bellevue Hospital.[16] He found a drop in both conditions, from 31.7 percent in 1910 to 5.8 percent in 1920, which he attributed to the good effects of Prohibition and the recognition of the "direct relation of the spirochaete to mental disease (Paresis)." The isolation of luetic nervous system infections from other mental conditions continued to be hailed as a boon to diagnosticians during the 1920s.

The public also felt relieved, for they too knew of cases of paresis and tabes that had silently and unexpectedly made their appearance among middle-aged men and women. The instinctive fear of this stealthy disease, perfectly embodied in Ibsen's *Ghosts,* maintained a strong hold on the public imagination. Now with scientific advances that fear could be quieted. H. L. Mencken, who was alert to all innovations in America, wrote, "Employment of that great diagnostic device [presumably the Wasserman test] was the discovery of thousands of cases of so-called mental disease . . . were actually victims of the small but extremely enterprising spirochaete pallida. . . . The news threw a bomb-shell into psychiatry."[17]

The "bomb-shell" included new treatments with the "magic bullet," Salvarsan (arsphenamine), in addition to the mercurial iodide standbys. There is a legend at old Bellevue Hospital that when arsphenamine reached New York, a syphilitic patient was given *one* injection with the expectation of a complete cure before a gathering of the entire faculty and student body. In any event, identification of the spirochete as the cause of a series of neuropsychiatric conditions brought the two opposing fields closer together. One example of the interpenetration of psychological thinking into the province of neurology appeared in a work on the mental dynamics of paretic patients by Stefan Hollas, a Hungarian psychiatrist, and his associate, Sandor Ferenczi, a psychoanalyst. Hollas and Ferenczi's paper, translated into English, appeared in the *Psychoanalytic Review* in 1925 and showed that the grandiosity and euphoria of the paretic, far from being a chance element in the disease, was a defensive reaction to the melancholia induced by "this calamitous disease" with its inevitable decline to death.[18] They prefaced their paper by remarking, "Hardly anyone has ventured to advance psychologic analysis to the psychic symptoms of General Paresis," and then went on to demonstrate in a careful study of several paretics that the dread fear of deterioration was converted within the psyche of the patient "to its opposite . . . the beginning of a new life." The megalomania resulting—"Every real loss is balanced by a rise in rank"—was embedded in delusions of grandeur that made the patient a king, a count, God, or a millionaire.

The entrance of a psychological aspect in organic disorders nourished the hope that somehow incurable diseases of the nervous system could be modified. Neurologists began to experiment with psychological treatment and gradually edged closer to the neuroses. Competition for patients became a factor in clinics and offices. Although the economic factor in neurological practice received no mention in scientific literature on the assumption that a fascination with the complex problems of localization sufficed the dedicated specialist, the subject *was* discussed in hospital cloakrooms. It was apparent that psychotherapy formed the base for a more durable practice than diagnostic work. Joseph Globus, Mount Sinai's gifted brain researcher, once related an occasion when, after his thorough neurological examination of a black Harlem resident, he was proffered four single dollars. Samuel Brock, professor of neurology at New York University and the author of a solid work on neurophysiology a generation ago, expressed the situation differently: "Practice is elusive," he said wistfully.[19] The economic struggle among nerve specialists for the increasing number of "nervous" patients requesting help depended upon the availability of effective treatment. And in truth, neurologists had few measures at their command. Although as Louis Casamajor pointed out, "American neurology was born of an attempt to treat psychoneurosis," its techniques were not too effective.[20] When neurosurgery evolved after World War I under the "aggressive leadership of Harvey Cushing," treatment became more effective: "They did something for their patients," Casamajor opined.[21]

Until neurosurgery developed some twenty years later, neurologists concentrated on localization of lesions and descriptions of clinical syndromes. This preoccupation did not go unnoticed. "You are more interested in diagnosis than etiology," Professor Anton Carlson, a Chicago neurophysiologist, scolded the members of the Chicago Neurological Society.[22] In defense of this and other attacks, Sidney Schwab in his presidential address before the American Neurological Association's annual meeting in 1921 asserted: "[The neurologist] is too readily impressed by . . . the traditional belief that some mysterious quality of mind is needed to venture into psychiatry. The psychiatric phase of neurology is a definite part of any neurologic activity."[23]

The real problem was treatment. In the so-called nerve clinics therapy was relatively routine. Bromides (usually triple bromides, for their presumed increased power), phenobarbital in the form of

Luminal or Veronal, arsenic as cacodylate, stomachics with minute quantities of strychnine—the ubiquitous Nux Vomica—and ferrous compounds were prescribed in profusion. The rationale for this type of therapeutics rested on George M. Beard's original theory of neurasthenia, the theory of "nerve exhaustion." It generally had been conceded that the nuclei of nerve cells shrank after exhaustion (or electrical excitation) and regained their normal function after rest and nutrition.[24] From this theory evolved the "rest cure," Weir Mitchell's insistence on nutrition, *Fat and Blood*,[25] and his widely read book, *Wear and Tear*,[26] as well as a warning of the neurologic cost of "restless living."

Other techniques involved the energizing effect of galvanic and faradic electricity. Electricity as a nervous system stimulant had been developed by Wilhelm Erb, a German pioneer in electrotherapy. In America George M. Beard became an enthusiastic proponent of it and wrote his *Medical and Surgical Uses of Electricity*, which became a standard text in America from its first publication as a 69-page monograph to its eighth edition of 599 pages in 1892.[27] Neurasthenic and depressed patients were treated for the next three decades with faradic and static electricity, usually delivered by a monster machine enclosed in a large glass case. Jelliffe recalled that during his student days in Europe, the "brutal electric spark treatment [was] orthodox in English and German clinics. . . . These patients never recovered."[28] As late as 1929, Richard Hutchings of the New York State hospital system recommended as "ideal" the following equipment in a physical therapy department: "low frequency generator, galvanic-sinusoidal machine, a static machine with at least 16 plates with insulating stool and wicker chair."[29] Equipment of this type remained in most physical therapy departments in general hospitals until about the late 1920s, a reminder, along with the Paquelin cautery, of more drastic therapy.

THE CHANGING STATUS OF NEUROLOGICAL THERAPY

Meanwhile neurologists in private practice enlarged their therapeutic techniques with hypnosis, suggestive treatment (Hippolyte-Marie Bernheim), and persuasion (Paul DuBois), including exploratory measures borrowed from psychoanalytical principles. The influence of the French school with its accent on *enfaiblessement* (restriction) of consciousness, the result of psychic exhaustion, was not entirely superseded. The term *psychasthenia* (Pierre Janet) carried the same message as neurasthenia (Beard), that is, a basic weakness of nerve function that called for strengthening measures. Thus in 1921, William Mallory adviced his fellow internists, "The present tendency is to speak of neurasthenia states or psychasthenic states, meaning increased irritability of the nervous system, with diminished capacity . . . Neurasthenia is an abnormal, imperfect, inadequate type of reaction expressive of auto-fixation."[30]

The psychasthenic concept still carried a connotation of mental weakness of some kind. In contrast, neurologists were beginning to feel comfortable with the psychodynamic ideas already accepted by most psychiatrists. For example, Isadore Coriat, a Boston psychoanalyst, wrote in 1924: "The informal and older descriptive psychiatry inaugurated by Kraepelin . . . is now rapidly drawing to a close. . . . Now [we are] interested in unconscious mechanisms of symptoms . . . behavior and utterances of psychotic patients."[31] In spite of this acceptance, younger men who tolerated, or even embraced, dynamic thinking were met headlong by neurologists who detested psychoanalysis.

The annual meeting of the American Neurological Society devoted much of its 1921 meeting to the rejection of this intrusive psychology. Dr. Charles K. Mills, a professor emeritus at the University of Pennsylvania, challenged the safety of psychoanalysis to potential patients as well as its lack of scientific validity. He inveighed against "the same evils as inflicted on the profession and community as . . . mystic and semi-mystic subjects, such as spiritism, Christian Science, divine healing, Corcesterism, evangelical healing, therapy at shrines like Lourdes."[32] At the same meeting, Professor Morton Prince of Harvard criticized the analytic school in milder tones, declaring that "[one] gives credit to the study of the 'dynamic sub-conscious' processess" in analysis, but no attention has been paid by Freud and his followers to "the great store of psychologic phenomena accumulated by experimental psychology."[33] In summary, Professor Prince concluded that psychoanalytic theory and therapy depended on "too elaborate, intricate and however ingenious, debatable interpretations of the subconscious. . . . [It is] more nearly a philosophy than a science." And Professor Mills agreed: "Psychoanalysis . . . [is] tending toward the discard. . . . It will lose its hold on the profession and the community in another generation."

Efforts to banish psychiatry from neurology proceeded for a decade. Older neurologists, revered for their clinical acumen and industry, continued to berate psychoanalysis, sometimes for reasons of scientific psychology, sometimes for pure pique. For example, in 1926 Bernard Sachs pointed to the "formidable array of clear-headed psychologists who refuse to accept [psychoanalysis]" and to the "two false conceptions . . . infantile sexuality and erotic dreams" that characterized Freudianism.[34] Sachs was incensed at the rising tide of analytic interest among the younger neurologists in his service at Mount Sinai Hospital. In an address at the New York Academy of Medicine, while describing his colleagueship with a certain young Viennese neurologist in the 1880s—"We sat together on the benches in Meynert's clinic"—he was startled to find that Freud's name had slipped from his memory. He stopped, tried to recall it, but could not. The audience chortled at this blatant proof of unconscious repression, the ultimate of *lapsus linguae.*

From the academic side the "formidable array of clear-headed psychologists" whom Sachs invoked, joined the fray. In 1920 Professor Knight Dunlap of Johns Hopkins University attacked the "Freudian system which appears to be fundamental[ly] antiscientific; with postulates of mysticism [and] a form of knowledge, consciousness, which is not yet conscious."[35] Professor William McDougall of Harvard in discussing Freud's primal horde theory against the father-figure theory concluded: "My verdict is not proven and wildly improbable . . . with all the peculiar Freudian assumptions on which it is based."[36] Diatribes of this type were answered by an occasional psychoanalyst. Karen Horney responded to Bernard Sachs's article "False Claims of the Psychoanalyst"[37] by averring that it "is riddled with *ad personam* arguments . . . obscuring rational thinking."[38]

Open opposition by leading neurologists continued. Frederick Peterson, a prominent and respected New York neuropsychiatrist, had welcomed Freud and Jung to America in their epoch making visit to Clark University in 1909. As professor of psychiatry at Columbia University he had advised one of his students, A. A. Brill, to visit Eugen Bleuler's "psychoanalytically inclined clinic at Burgholzli, rather than those in Paris or Munich with Kraepelin" according to Clarence Oberndorf.[39] As the years passed and Peterson observed patients treated by psychoanalysis, he too joined the detractors on the issue of treatment success. In a 1919 article titled "Credulity and Cures," Peterson reviewed some irregular treatment methods in vogue and faulted analysts for "bad results with young people . . . even permanent insanity."[40] Although he knew Freud and Jung personally and was aware of their discoveries, his negative position became stronger in time. An editorial in the *Journal of the American Medical Association* in 1933 quoted a letter written by Peterson saying "[psychoanalysis] is a voodoo religion characterized by obscene rites and human sacrifices . . . [that is] unfortunate victims of psychoanalysis."[41] The editorial writer tried to soften the impact of this denunciation: "It would be folly," he wrote, "to deny that the work of Sigmund Freud is a fundamental contribution. . . . It would be equally fallacious to assert that it is an unmixed blessing."

The seemingly everlasting wrangling between the organic and psychologic groups lasted through the 1930s. While hard-line neurologists turned away from Freudian psychiatry, most organicists listened with respect to Adolf Meyer, who throughout his career pleaded for a commonsense view of nervous and mental troubles, while faintly acknowledging Freudianism. "The nightmare of neuropsychiatric dilemma has no place," declared Meyer.[42] He counseled, "One learns to subordinate the exaggerated contrast of mind and body, and to speak of reactions of the internal or visceral organs, the nervous segmental and suprasegmental organs and functions as such, or as parts of the reactions of the cerebrally integrated person." Some neurologists, however, stuck to their convictions. Stanley Cobb, a Boston neurologist, maintained that "wherever brain functions there is organic change. . . . Organic change takes place whenever a person has a thought. . . . The slang terms 'organic or functional' are meaningless."[43]

The controversy equally involved economic and professional conflicts. Most nerve specialists of the time treated both neurological and psychiatric cases in office practice. Textbook writers included chapters on neuroses and psychoses in neurological texts until the late 1920s. Israel Wechsler, professor of neurology at Columbia University, not only added a chapter on psychiatric problems to his well-regarded *A Textbook of Clinical Neurology*[44] but also wrote a book titled *The Neuroses*[45] two years after the first edition of his text. An urbane gentleman, later chief of the neurological service at Mount Sinai Hospital, Wechsler used to say smilingly that he "bootlegged psychiatry." As patients became more knowledgeable about newer treatments for emotional troubles, the profession felt it needed to define the two fields more precisely.

At the New York Academy of Medicine, meetings were devoted to the question of whether neuropsychiatry was a valid hyphenization or whether each specialty should stand alone. At one of these meetings Dr. Sachs said, "No one is able to draw a hard and fast line between neurology and psychiatry. . . . We are all neuropsychiatrists." Ramsay Hunt of the Neurological Institute, a man of dignity and measured speech, recalled the important neurological influences in psychiatry: "The ideal psychiatrist of the future will be a neuro-psychiatrist." In a prophetic vein, he added, "Who knows what may happen in a few decades in the field of chemistry in relation to cells in the brain. . . . [It may] build up a new psychiatry." Israel Strauss agreed: "We must connect the functional and organic." After much discussion a committee headed by Vernon Branham reported that they found the term "neuropsychiatry" valid and honorable.[46] In spite of the neuropsychiatric dialectic, the neurological output in the United States during the 1920s was enormous. Clinical and pathological studies of encephalitis, multiple sclerosis, syphilis of the central nervous system, brain and spinal cord tumors, viral infections, neuralgias and neuritis, demyelinating diseases, myopathies, and congenital deformities filled the journals. At the same time occasional articles on psychiatry, especially those dealing with dementia praecox, were given ample space in neurological journals. Even as late as 1931, the *Archives of Neurology and Psychiatry* reprinted the 1929 proceedings of the German Neurological Society, as well as the proceedings of the New York, Chicago, Philadelphia,

Boston, and San Francisco societies.[47] As Israel Wechsler commented in his textbook on neurology, "Up to the end of the 19th century, America took more from Europe than it gave. . . . [Still] beginning with the 20th century, there has been a tremendous burst of activity in neurology in America."[48]

While neurology as a clinical subject was developing, the more precise aspects of the field—neurophysiology and microscopic analysis of diseased cerebral tissue—were progressing even more rapidly. Additionally, discoveries of the English scientists, Sherrington, Starling, and Fulton in America, of nerve impulses and their chemical and physiological properties and functions, became basic to an understanding of clinical neurology.

EDUCATION IN NEUROPSYCHIATRY

Pleas for better training in neurology and psychiatry had been voiced for years before they became an actuality. In 1914 William Graves of Saint Louis University in a paper titled "Some Factors Tending Towards Adequate Instruction in Nervous and Mental Disease" concluded by asking: "Does the standard medical curriculum . . . and do medical schools allot to neurology and psychiatry, time and place proportionate to the importance of these branches?"[49] World War I experiences pushed the need for training in neuropsychiatry to the fore. By 1917 Edward Strecker, a consultant to the War Department, had responded to the need by developing a six-week course held at hospitals throughout the country: Boston Psychopathic, Mendocino Hospital in California, New York Neurological Institute, Philadelphia General, Phipps Institute at Johns Hopkins, University of Michigan Psychopathic, and Saint Elizabeths Hospital in Washington, D.C.[50] For the first time the focus was on psychiatry rather than neurology. Even after the war, the earlier momentum carried the planning forward. Henry Bunker noted that "several chairs in the Medical Psychology were established by the end of the war."[51] A few years later, John Whitehorn, while reviewing research departments in leading universities, stated: "Training in psychiatry at the University of Michigan, Harvard University, and Johns Hopkins . . . [has] produced more psychiatrists than any other medical schools."[52]

In less prestigious schools, teachings in the mental sciences remained skimpy.

At the college level, preparation for understanding the neurosciences—a term not yet coined—was nonexistent. Liberal arts college courses in psychology did little to prepare a premedical student for clinical neuropsychiatry. Departments of psychology used texts that emphasized physiological psychology with diagrams detailing reflex pathways between cortex and peripheral nerves that bore only a shadowy resemblance to mental ills. Discussions of hysteria and phobias, multiple personalities, and the coconscious of Morton Prince, enlivened psychology courses, but academe was wary of admitting psychoanalytical concepts into the classroom. At the University of Cincinnati such esoterica was discussed more, curiously enough, in classes on English literature than in classes on psychology. Premedical students eschewed such intangible subjects as psychology. But because of a tropism that I felt directed me toward psychiatry, I "camped" (an "in" expression at the time) around the psychology department, typed a manuscript on the psychology of music for Professor Charles Diserens, and performed a few chores for the department heads, Professors B. B. Breese and Talbot.

The tropism theory, which was originated by Jacques Loeb of the Rockefeller Institute, had been advanced to explain the drives, instincts, and impulsions of human beings on a mechanical basis. If I had known of unconscious identification at that time, I might have recognized that my tropism for nervous and mental areas rested on my mother's early fascination with *hystérie*, which dated from her days as a student nurse at the Moscow University and reflected her admiration for her French professor of midwifery, who was reputed to be a *morphiniste*. (Russian students had a particular admiration for the French in prerevolution days.) In any event, my predilection for nervous and mental areas extended to neuroanatomy when I attained the freshman medical class. Our professor of anatomy, one Dr. Knower, seemed to sense this impulsion, for he suggested that I pursue a special research project that involved dissecting out the cervical sympathetic ganglia in a cadaver. Presented with a preserved head and neck of a Negro male that was set on a block of wood in a small room near the laboratory, I was left in the gathering darkness of a winter's afternoon to accomplish my task, which went beyond the regular class work. As the students left for the day, I started my eerie project alone, a textbook propped on the table, the imperturbable cadaver's head facing me. As the work progressed, I became unnerved, aware that I was not sure I knew what I was doing or why I was doing it. Within a few weeks I abandoned the project to the muted amusement of the professor.

But the tropism, if that what it was, had not been quieted. During the next year, while locked into physiology, pathology, histology, and other routine studies, I had the opportunity to work as a night orderly in Cincinnati General Hospital. After a few months duty in the operating room as flunky to the scrub nurses and surgeons, I was assigned to the evening-to-morning shift in the psychopathic pavilion. Here both psychiatric and neurological cases were housed. My task was simply to watch the disturbed patients and report to the intern on duty. I watched confused seniles, languishing suicidal subjects, aphasic paralytics, melancholics, and a case of spotted fever (meningitis). With a growing sense of bewilderment, I could only retreat to studies of more comprehensive medical subjects in preparation for the next day's classes. The daily classes, however, provided glimpses that promised order out of the chaos I witnessed on the ward. Our professor of biochemistry, Albert P. Mathews, included in his biochemistry text a chapter on the brain, dramatically titled "The Master Tissue of the Body." That in itself was intriguing, even esoteric, in contrast to other subjects we studied. Indeed, the biochemistry department exuded a special aura. While Professor Mathews lectured in a tweed jacket and plus fours, the very image of a British sportsman-scientist, his associate, Shiro Tashiro, a small, intense Japanese, continued his earlier researches, demonstrating the chemical nature of the nerve impulse. The aura of science clung to Tashiro. Like Hideyo Noguchi, his countryman, Professor Tashiro was capable of intense concentration. It was said of Noguchi that when he was developing pure cultures of the *Treponema pallidum* in the laboratory around 1911, he worked for days at a time without seeing the outside world. So, too, Tashiro in the biochemistry laboratory would thoughtfully listen to and gather four or five questions at a time from as many students and then serially unload the answers to the questioners.

When I returned to New York for the last two years of medicine at Long Island College Hospital, some of the romance of medical research faded. The school, located in downtown Brooklyn and fashioned on the old British model of a college hospital, became the precursor of the present State University of New York, Downstate Medical Center. At the time it conveyed little of the spirit of a university medical center. Its role was to turn out doctors who would pass the state board examinations and then hang out a shingle, tend multiparous mothers, feverish babies, and do what was known as "bread and butter" minor surgery in the office. To answer their practical medical needs, which were dedicated to obstetrics, surgery, and pediatrics, little attention was paid to neurology and less to psychiatry. Our neurology professor, Dr. Browning, a sprightly older man who with his goatee and wing collar dressed in a manner reminiscent of Weir Mitchell of post-Civil War fame, demonstrated how one could test pupillary reflexes with a head mirror and a shaft of light, check abdominal reflexes with a toothpick, and elicit knee jerks with the back of one's hand. Dr. Browning wisked through a few tests, discussed syphilis of the nervous system and tetanus in a lively, anecdotal way, and after two lectures turned us over to his assistant, Dr. Osmond Perkins. Dutifully Dr. Perkins demonstrated a variety of pathological gaits in actual patients and in caricature with little detail of pathology or therapeutics. Similarly, the psychiatric instructors demonstrated dementia praecox and manic-depressive patients at the Brooklyn State Hospital as isolated experiences.

Actually the larger departments at the Kings County Hospital contained active neurological services, especially the neurosurgical service under Jeffrey Browder. Students in the period from 1924 to 1926, however, had no contact with this area of activity. Indeed, the atmosphere was curiously parochial (the trustees had been trying to affiliate with Princeton University without success). Clinical material was conveyed chiefly through lectures and added to by the enormous pile of lecture notes our student leader brought to the nightly study group. We memorized as our bible, Osler's *Textbook of Medicine.* It was a bookish type of learning that carried a faintly European overtone. In the lecture hall, students sat in steeply tiered seats, straining to hear the lecturer in the pit. The scene was reminiscent of a medieval picture of neophytes raptly witnessing a dissection by Vesalius of Padua in the sixteenth century.

University medical schools fared little better with respect to neuropsychiatry. Louis Casamajor, reminiscing about his student days at Columbia's College of Physicians and Surgeons prior to 1920, recalled "the students got three or four clinics in psychiatry during the fourth year. We did not learn a thing but we enjoyed the show."[53] Although Cornelius Wholey, writing in the *Journal of the American Medical Association* in 1930, noted the paucity of psychiatric education in the medical schools—"Many medical schools do not emphasize the importance of mental factors in disease . . ."—psychiatric teaching at Long Island improved at this time.[54] Frank L. Babbott, then president of Long Island Medical College, strengthened the psychiatric department by inviting Alfred Adler to become visiting professor of medical psychology in 1932 and by inviting William White, an early graduate (1891) to speak on *The Place of Psychiatry in General Medicine* at the annual alumni dinner in May 1935.[55] Later, during the 1940s, Sandor Lorand, an eminent psychoanalyst, was appointed to the faculty of Downstate Medical Center, the successor to Long Island Medical Center. In general, psychiatry in most medical schools throughout the country remained a mystical field for the medical student until World War II.

Nevertheless, the main subjects were well covered and few students failed the New York State Board examinations. During their senior year, students were externed at various hospitals, some at such first-rate institutions as Brooklyn Hospital, Brooklyn Jewish Hospital, and Greenpoint Hospital. I drew an assignment to the local Holy Family Hospital in Red Hook, an old red-bricked building reminiscent of what might be encountered in Liverpool, England. There I made rounds with the interns, dressed sores, became familiar with pneumonias, indolent varicose ulcers, and wounds inflicted on long-suffering wives by the hands of their bibulous husbands. On ambulance duty the driver introduced me to fecundity and easy death, the price of living in the infamous

Red Hook district of Brooklyn. Exsanguinated women, brought to the hospital to remedy a miscarriage, alternated with babies dying of the "summer complaint." Sickness and despair were accepted; a "cross to bear": "Tis the will of God" whispered the sisters who tended the sick.

Neurology for the Resident

Meanwhile, progress at leading neurological institutes proceeded apace. Under Frederick Tilney and Henry Riley, the New York Neurological Institute became part of the Columbia-Presbyterian Hospital complex on Washington Heights. Bellevue's neurological service under the leadership of Foster Kennedy and Mount Sinai's department headed by Bernard Sachs, who was succeeded by Israel Strauss, became recognized teaching institutions for residents.

My entrance into the universe of neurology as a resident on the Mount Sinai Hospital service followed a rotating internship at that institution. The atmosphere there was unique in its devotion to scientific medicine; a spirit of discipline and a hierarchical Teutonic system controlled and educated the staff. German and Viennese medicine reigned supreme, especially in neurology, although the penumbra of French and British neurology also illuminated the clinical landscape. At Mount Sinai, the chief of each service ruled his staff. Orders were transmitted through a chain of command, from chief to associate to assistant to resident and finally to the intern. On medical rounds opinions and comments came down in this order. In surgery the intern got no closer to the body on the operating table than "pulling third retractor" or snipping suture ends if the intern was considered experienced or gifted enough. The attitudes of the lower echelon on the house staff were reverential. On the medical side, Emmanuel Libman and B. S. Oppenheimer ranked high. In surgery A. A. Berg was almost deified. The flavor of Germanic medical autocracy was supported by such men as Bella Schick in pediatrics, the originator of the Schick diphtheria test, Burril Crohn of Crohn's disease, Bernard Sachs of Tay-Sachs disease. The house staff lived, ate, and slept medicine with a dedication suggestive of Albert Schweitzer's reverence for life.

When I became a resident, the chief of neurology, Israel Strauss, had just succeeded Bernard Sachs. Sachs, equipped with the obligatory goatee and vest with white piping, made an imposing figure, the epitome of the "gentleman neurologist," so-called because he rarely became involved with noisome things like abdominal contents, sputum, or running sores. Under Dr. Strauss, some of the ponderousness evaporated. A vigorous, incisive leader, he was deeply interested in both research and the training of his staff. Here the spirit was more democratic. Everyone of the staff of the neurology department became involved in the monthly department meetings at which cases from the wards were analyzed and no diagnostic possibility was left unexplored. The associate staff joined the discussion; E. D. Friedman, professor at New York University, Moses Keschner, a medicolegal expert, and others expounded their clinical opinions. Like a Supreme Court justice, Dr. Strauss logically narrowed the possibilities of clinical diagnosis, aided at times by the neuropathological demonstrations of Joseph Globus.[56] Dr. Globus, a Russian who looked more like a freedom fighter in a Balkan state than a pathologist, had done outstanding work in delineating the cellular structure of the *glioblastoma multiforme*, a lethal type of brain tumor.

Globus and Strauss had discovered the tumor, now called *spongioblastoma,* as a result of their coordinated clinical-pathologic study.[57] Globus had a flair for the dramatic, which made the neuro-pathological conferences unforgettable. On one occasion, as he demonstrated on a slide an enlarged spongioblast that had grown expansive and destructive, he pointed to the solitary nucleus and described it as "a Cyclops with one eye in the forehead." Indeed, neuropathology by the late 1920s had become a vital aspect of neurology. The findings in the neuropathological laboratory were depended on as the final arbiters of diagnostic skill. Not only at Mount Sinai but also at institutes in Europe and elsewhere in this country, laboratories were carrying out gross and microscopic analyses of brain tissue; Golgi, Bielshowsky, Von Giesen, Weigert-Pal techniques brought to light the intricate structure of nervous tissue and the products of its decay.

Residency on the neurological service provided an "open sesame" to a field I barely knew existed. During the year, I examined 441 cases of the most varied types. In my notes I counted 46 patients with central nervous system lues, 27 cases of encephalitis, 76 brain tumors, 68 of which set down as psychic disturbances, numerous cases of radiculitis, neuritis, meningitis, multiple sclerosis, Raynaud's disease, spondylosis rhizomyelique, and 13 that were placed in the category of "rare conditions." Each examined case received a review by the attending neurologist who suggested various procedures that were entrusted to the resident staff: spinal punctures, measurements of fluid pressure, peripheral field examinations, pneumoencephalograms through the spinal route— even cisterna punctures—and epidural injections for sciatica. Occasionally on grand rounds, foreign visitors, once Professor J. A. Sicard of Paris and once several Japanese neurologists, were given over to me and my assistant resident for a tour of the service. Beyond this, we were privileged to "pull third retractor" or tie off sutures with the neurosurgeon Charles Elsberg, a pioneer in spinal surgery, which then was still in its early stages. To be allowed to assist him at the operating table gave one a feeling of witnessing a pioneer in medicine as he cautiously worked in this obscure area.

The main emphasis during my residency, however, was on diagnosis and localization of lesions. Treatment, aside from surgery, was minimal since the field contained more unknowns than knowns. To become acquainted with this vast array of diagnoses, both common and esoteric, we had a further resource, the Montefiore Hospital for Chronic Diseases, which was located in the northern reaches of the Bronx. It functioned as a museum of such living rareties as Little's disease, dystonias, chronic choreas, striatal disorders, muscular dystrophies, and glandular problems. Monthly conferences at Montefiore filled out the panoply of rare conditions that are the preoccupation of clinicians and embryo neurologists. This depository of flailing limbs and distorted bodies furnished Phillip Goodhart, and Charles Davison (before he deserted neuropathology for psychoanalysis) with rich material for papers on complex striatal diseases.[58] Indeed, the search for rare diseases fitted the tradition at Mount Sinai. It was the so-called *Arbeit*, the accepted pathway to medical notice, if not fame. Research held high rank in that scientific atmosphere.

Luckily, such a case presented itself to me in the form of a four-year-old child who had been admitted on the child neurology service with marked exophthalmus, a history of excessive thirst, and diminutive height. The child presented a rare combination of diabetes insipidus, marked exopthalmus, and soft areas in the skull vault. With Dr. Louis Hausman, assistant professor of neuro-anatomy at Cornell Medical School, our *Arbeit* became an analysis of this unusual bony dystocia of the sphenoid bone involving the hypophysis, hence the diabetes insipidus and exopthalmus. Our paper, which included the case among the dystrophy group, was published in the *Archives of Neurology and Psychiatry* in 1929.[59] It developed, however, that the case belonged to the Schueller-Hand-Christian syndrome, a type of lipoid deterioration of the cranial bones.[60] With this paper a vast neurologic literature opened to my view.

A Neurological Feast

Reading the *Archives* each month became an ordained duty that was supplemented by attendance at meetings at the New York Academy of Medicine. This was a clinical exercise that outdid the promise of the Allegemeine Krankenhause in Vienna or Queen's Square Hospital in London, at that time two Meccas for young neurologists. The academy was a unique institution. Its library was comprehensive, the reading rooms even dramatic and elegant. The back room containing rare books was often the private pre-serve of Smith Ely Jelliffe. Seated at a table loaded with books, he ran through his monthly book reviews for the *Journal of Nervous and Mental Disease*. The journal, which was his publication venture into the new fields of psychoanalysis and neuropsychiatry, became a mirror image of Jelliffe's personality.

Jelliffe himself was a unique character. Broadly read, articulate, at home in Greek and Latin classics, which he often quoted in society discussions, his roots were deep in America. When I visited him in his office on West Fifty-fifth Street, I ascended a brownstone stairway and entered through a door adorned with a flowered glass pane. His office, lined with books, contained a sarcophagus-like couch (presumably similar to the one Freud used) and an enormous chair from which he delivered his opinions in a firm, clear voice. His ironic wit, which was combined with an encyclopedic knowledge, was equally evident in book reviews in the journal, for they were written with a keen appreciation of both scientific

reliability and possible cant. In writing of Arnold Gesell's innovative *The Mental Growth of the Pre-School Child* in 1925,
Jelliffe commented, "A book of transcendent interest. . . . Stanley
Hall would have welcomed such a study. . . . Yet so rigid. . . . The
apotheosis of science on ice!"[61] Of Louis Berman's *Glands Regulating Personality,* Jelliffee wrote "hooey of the cheapest kind,"
and of Morris Fishbein's critique of psychoanalysis in his book
Frauds in Medicine, he said, "[Fishbein] wrote with incomprehensible inaccuracy." But Fishbein was not to be vanquished. In his
next book, *New Medical Follies,* which appeared in 1927, Fishbein
characterized psychoanalysis as "one of the greatest sources of
controversy to appear on the medical scene" and then stated in
his autobiography, "Dr Jelliffe . . . willing to accept statements
made in every field but his own . . . was intolerant of criticism
of the special areas of Freudian techniques."[62]

Unlike the growing band of European psychoanalysts residing
in New York with a specific loyalty to Freudian metapsychology,
Jelliffe maintained a keen interest in neurological lesions and
their symbolic meaning. For example, in his elaborate study of
post-encephalitic respiratory disorders, he pointed to the similarity
between organically induced symptoms and psychogenic respiratory
disorders.[63] Sensing a relationship between tics and dystonias in
cases of degenerative nervous system disease and the peculiar
postures and movements of the hysteric, he postulated that
unconscious conflicts could mimic involuntary movements similar
to those of organic brain disease. Odd tics, particularly oculogyric
crises, which were just beginning to appear in the wake of the 1918-
1920 sleeping sickness epidemic, contained elements startlingly like
those of catatonia or major hysteria. This early psychosomatic
relationship, published in 1932,[64] was reviewed by Lawrence Kubie
in the *Psychoanalytic Quarterly* as an "unscientific" effort.[65]
Kubie, who had been a neurophysiologist at Columbia before
becoming an analyst, first at Yale University and then at Shepard
and Enoch Pratt near Baltimore, Maryland, objected to Jelliffe's
"retreating into the world of classical erudition . . . to legitimate
efforts at anatomical localization . . . [where] one is bemused by
the incomprehensible distinction . . . between organic and psychic
processes." Behind Kubie's criticism of Jelliffe's lack of scientific

criteria, lay a stylistic irritation with the "frequent use of colloquial, semi-obscene or facetious slang expressions" to which Jelliffe pleaded "no contest." This minor skirmish may have been the reason for Jelliffe's obscene characterization of Kubie when the latter denied by one vote Paul Schilder's membership in the New York Psychoanalytic Association (see p. 89).

In any event, this episode, as well as others, branded Jelliffe as an eclectic, and at this time, loyalty to one system of therapy dominated the scene. Freud had set the tone in his *New Introductory Lectures:* "The circumstance that the structure of psychoanalysis . . . already possesses a unified organization from which one cannot select elements according to one's whims."[66] The issue of eclecticism (using the best of every system for the benefit of the patient) received a negative imprimatur and made Jelliffe's stance suspect among psychoanalysts. Oberndorf in his *History of Psychoanalysis in America,* recalled that when Freud met Jelliffe in Vienna in 1921, the latter's "eclectic Americanism" brought him into "slight disfavor" in the master's eyes.[67] Jelliffe was acutely aware of this. In his reminiscences, *Glimpses of a Freudian Odyssey,* published in 1933, he related how the *Psychoanalytic Review* opened its pages with a contribution by Jung instead of Freud, since "we were not then . . . oriented to the developing differences within the inner circle. . . . At all events the *Review* has gone its way with a certain eclecticism . . . justified in this country."[68]

Forceful in his discussions, Jelliffe could make startling, newsworthy statements at medical meetings. On one occasion at the Academy of Medicine, I and a large audience of New York psychiatrists heard him explain Irving Berlin's extraordinary sense of syncopation as due to his mother's irregular heartbeat (auricular fibrillation) during her pregnancy. The story appeared on the front page of the *New York Times,* but it later developed he had made the same comment, according to George Daniels, years before at the 1923 session of the American Neurological Association.[69] At another time, as an expert witness in the celebrated case of Harry K. Thaw, the millionaire playboy who shot Stanford White in what was known as "the murder of the century," Jelliffe testified to Thaw's insanity and sued for the unpaid fee of $10,000 after

Thaw's acquittal and subsequent incarceration at the Matteawan State Hospital for the Criminally Insane. The murderer's escape from the institution to Canada gave rise to the phrase, now part of Americana, "to get away with murder." The story of the suit again reached the *Times,* but Jelliffe reaped only press coverage. In reviewing Jelliffe's early assays into holistic medicine, Daniels commented, "Jelliffe enjoys bold statements . . . many are brilliant, some overshoot the mark."[70]

His boldness might have been called a species of "imaginative psychiatry;" that is, a slighting of strict logic for an artistic perception of the whole. Karl Menninger recalled at the commemoration of Jelliffe's thirty-fifth year as editor of the *Journal of Nervous and Mental Disease* in 1938 that the latter had once written him: "In science one must choose between the absolutely safe but entirely sterile on the one hand, and on the other, of having courage to think beyond one's facts."[71] It was this courage that Menninger noted, when as a "Kansas boy," fresh from a residency and on a *Wanderjahr* in the East, he had been befriended by Jelliffe in Manhattan. As Doctor Karl recalled the contact in 1920, "Jelliffe talked incessantly about psycho-analysis. . . . It was astonishing to me. . . . [It had] not been so in Boston, not so in Baltimore, but Ah, New York."[72] For myself, Jelliffe's maverick spirit was enlivening. Years after his death, I had an uncanny experience when sitting with a patient in Sacramento, early in my settling in the then psychiatrically cold atmosphere of Northern California—Jelliffe and White's textbook suddenly fell onto the floor from a number of other books undisturbed on the shelf. A year later the same spectral experience was repeated and not since; and no explanation I could conjure up was ever satisfactory!

NEUROLOGICAL ADVANCES

A major contribution of this colorful neuropsychiatrist was the establishment of the Nervous and Mental Monograph series with William A. White. The series published Breuer and Freud's pioneer *Studies in Hysteria,* as translated by A. A. Brill. Their list of publications contained many of the fundamental writings of the period, varying from William White's *Foundations of*

Psychiatry through Freud's *Three Contributions to the Sexual Theory,* Edward Kempf's *The Autonomic Functions and the Personality,* and Paul Schilder's *Brain and Personality.* There was scarcely a seminal thinker in the field who did not find a place in Jelliffe and White's publishing list. The *Journal of Nervous and Mental Disease,* edited by Jelliffe and succeeded by the *Psychoanalytic Review,* spread the gospel of analytic thinking among neurologists.

Stimulating as the neurological literature was, the monthly meetings of clinical subdivisions at the academy were even more energizing. Academy sections on ophthalmology, medicine, otolaryngology were important, but the *pièce de résistance* was the section on neurology and psychiatry. The discussions that followed each presentation varied, as did the papers, from cortical decortication through intoxication with carbon dioxide by Israel Wechsler to analysis of the best method for sectioning the trigeminal nerve for tic doloreaux by Byron Stookey, the neurosurgeon. His intrepid operation was answered by Dr. Dandy of Baltimore whose work in the same field yielded differing results. Discussions were serious, spirited and sometimes acrimonious, as the men spoke out of their experience. For five years after I entered the neurological field, I attended the section meetings at the academy with the devotion of an opera buff.

The material covered every aspect of neurology—Parkinsonism, dystonias, subacute combined sclerosis (pernicious anemia), central nervous system infections, brain tumors, head injuries, syringomyelia, Raynaud's disease, epilepsy, cerebral vascular lesions. At one meeting, Foster Kennedy, chief of the Bellevue neurological service and a professor at Cornell, with his clipped English speech and British locutions crossed swords with Israel Strauss, intent on logical explanations in the diagnosis of a brain tumor; at another, Ramsay Hunt, a venerable neurologist, talked of his discovery of neuralgia of the geniculate ganglion; Walter Timme related the course of an endocrine problem; Temple Fay of Philadelphia discoursed on his ketogenic diet for epileptics. Men from other centers made their appearance: Samuel Orton of Iowa described dyslexia as due to strephosymbolia, an inability to form symbols for language; Dandy of Baltimore displayed pneumography and ventriculography; Wilder Penfield of McGill University, Pierce Bailey of Chicago, Harvey Cushing of Boston spoke on their neurosurgical innovations. The *Archives* covered these and a host of other contributions by individual workers, producing a rich harvest in neurology, neuropathology, and neurosurgery.[73]

Bernard Hart pointed out the common stages of growth in science: (1) collection of data, (2) description and classification, (3) interpretation and application.[74] It can be said that the period of the early 1930s fulfilled the second stage. Besides outstanding men—W. G. Spiller and Edward Strecker of Philadelphia, Abraham Myerson, William Lennox, and Stanley Cobb of Boston, Charles Neymann and Loyal Davis of Chicago—there were many whose contributions filled the pages of specialty journals. Those in the New York area whom I worked under or heard in conferences included Michael Osnato, chief of clinical neurology at the Post-Graduate Hospital; Armando Ferraro, neuropathologist at the psychiatric institute on Ward's Island and later in the Columbia Medical Center; Leo M. Davidoff, a student of Harvey Cushing, a neurosurgeon active in developing pneumoencephalography; Walter Timme, an endocrinologist; and Henry Riley of Columbia University. The mention of these neurological giants floods the memory with images of lesser lights. But there were no lesser lights; whether they improved diagnoses by added bits of clinical detail or hazarded a new treatment technique in written form or at a clinical conference, they were diligent, dedicated workers. Devotees of the expanding horizon of neurology—men like Louis Casamajor of the Neurological Institute who described "brain fever," a resurrected diagnosis of earlier days in a series of cases that began in 1935[75]—enlivened the often obscure problems facing the neurologist. It was truly a Golden Age of American neurology.

Inevitably, psychiatric concerns vied for attention. Near the end of the third decade, psychiatric writings began to fill the pages of the *Archives* and the *Journal of Nervous and Mental Disease*. At one 1930 meeting of the New York Neurological Society, Lawson Lowrey and David Levy, child guidance experts, discussed problems among abnormal children.[76] Oswald Boltz, a senior psychiatrist at the Manhattan State Hospital, read a paper on unconscious homosexual factors precipitating schizophrenia.[77] At another meeting, Pierce Clark, one of the older neurologists, read a paper on the epileptical convulsion as a symbolic masturbatory act to the visible consternation of the audience.[78]

The viability of psychiatry had been established. Internists accepted medical psychology as a valid part of medicine. The oncoming generation of neurologists joined a small band of neurosurgeons or drifted into neuropsychiatry with an accent on psychotherapy. In the main, psychiatry as an independent discipline moved away from neurology. In time, the Cinderella of medicine bypassed the queen of the medical sciences.

NOTES

1. Adolf Meyer, *Collected papers,* ed. F. Ebaugh (Baltimore, Md.: Johns Hopkins Press, 1951), 3:546.

2. Weir Mitchell, "Address before the Fiftieth Meeting of the American Medico-Psychological Association," *Proceedings,* 1894, p. 101.

3. Walter Channing, "Some Remarks on the Address Delivered at the American Medico-Psychological Association Meeting by Weir Mitchell," *American Journal of Insanity* 51 (October 1894): 170.

4. Louis Casamajor, "Notes for an Intimate History of Neurology and Psychiatry in America," *Journal of Nervous and Mental Disease* 98 no. 6 (December 1943): 600.

5. D. E. Denny-Brown, "The Changing Pattern of Neurologic Medicine," *New England Journal of Medicine* 246 no. 22 (May 29, 1952): 839-46.

6. Franz Nissl, quoted in A. Meyer, "A Few Trends in Modern Psychiatry," *Psychology Bulletin* 1 (1904): 217.

7. Erwin Stengel, "The Origin and Status of Dynamic Psychiatry," *British Journal of Medical Psychology* 27 (1954): 193-200.

8. F. W. Langdon, "Neurological Progress and Prospects," *Journal of the American Association* (hereafter *JAMA*) 41, no. 3 (January 10, 1903): 145.

9. Albert Barrett, "Syphilitic Psychosis Associated with Manic-Depressive Psychosis, Symptoms and Course," *JAMA* 67 no. 23 (December 2, 1916): 1639.

10. B. P. Thom, "Tertiary Syphilis Psychosis Other Than Paresis," *American Journal of Insanity* 78 (April 1921): 503.

11. Smith E. Jelliffe and William A. White, *Diseases of the Nervous System, A Textbook of Neurology and Psychiatry,* 4th ed., rev. (Philadelphia: Lea & Febriger, 1923), p. 752.

12. Ibid., p. 730.

13. Ibid., p. 845.

14. Ibid., p. 752.

15. William Malamud, "The History of Psychiatric Therapies," in *One Hundred Years of American Psychiatry,* ed. J. K. Hall (New York: Columbia University Press, 1944), p. 302.

16. George H. Kirby, "Alcohol and Syphilis as Causes of Mental Disease," *JAMA* 76 no. 16 (April 16, 1921): 1062.

17. Henry L. Mencken, *Prejudices,* 2d series (New York: Alfred A. Knopf, 1920), p. 166.

18. Stefan Hollas and S. Ferenczi, "Psychoanalysis and the Psychiatric Disorder of General Paralysis," trans. G. Barnes and G. Keil, *Psychoanalytic Review* 12, no. 1 (January 1925): 88, 205.

19. Personal communication, 1928.

20. Casamajor, "Notes for an Intimate History," p. 600.

21. Ibid., p. 607.

22. Anton Carlson, "Comment," *Archives of Neurology and Psychiatry* 6 (September 1921): 259.

23. Sidney Schwab, "The Neurologic Dilemma," *Archives of Neurology and Psychiatry* 6 (September 1921): 259.

24. George M. Beard, "Neurasthenia or Nervous Exhaustion," *Medical and Surgical Journal* 3 (April 1869): 368.

25. Silas Weir Mitchell, *Fat and Blood, An Essay on the Treatment of Certain Forms of Neurasthenia and Hysteria* (Philadelphia: J. B. Lippincott, 1877).

26. Silas Weir Mitchell, *Wear and Tear, or Hints for the Overworked* (Philadelphia: J. B. Lippincott, 1871).

27. George M. Beard and A. D. Rockwell, *Medical and Surgical Uses of Electricity,* 8th ed. (New York: Wood, 1892).

28. Smith E. Jelliffe, "Deaths of M. Allen Starr and Jos. F. Babinski," *JAMA* 100 no. 2 (January 14, 1933): 134.

29. Richard Hutchings "Organization of a Physical Therapy Department in a State Hospital," *Psychiatric Quarterly,* 3 (1929): 203.

30. William J. Mallory, "The Neurasthenic Patient and the Internist," *JAMA* 76 no. 12 (March 19, 1921): 788.

31. Isadore Coriat, "Progress in Psychiatry," *Boston Medical and Surgical Journal* 191, no. 11 (September 1924): 499.

32. Charles K. Mills, "Some Theoretical and Some Practical Aspects

of Psychoanalysis," *Archives of Neurology and Psychiatry* 6 (December 21, 1921): 608.

33. Morton Prince, "A Critique of Psychoanalysis," *Archives of Neurology and Psychiatry* 6 (December 21, 1921): 608.

34. Bernard Sachs, *The Normal Child and How to Keep it Normal in Mind and Morals* (New York: Paul Hoeber Co., 1926), pp. 72, 94.

35. Knight Dunlap, *Mysticism, Freudianism, and Scientific Psychology* (St. Louis: C. V. Mosby Co., 1920), p. 89.

36. William McDougall, in *Problems of Personality,* ed. Maefie Campbell et al. (New York: Harcourt, Brace Co., 1925), 267.

37. Bernard Sachs, "False Claims of Psychoanalysis," *American Journal of Psychiatry* 12 (January 1933): 725.

38. Karen Horney, Letter to the Editor, *JAMA* 100 no. 15 (April 15, 1933): 1196.

39. Clarence P. Oberndorf, *A History of Psychoanalysis in America* (New York: Grune & Stratton, 1953), p. 53.

40. Frederick Peterson, "Credulity and Cures," *JAMA* 73 (December 1919).

41. Editorial, *JAMA* 100, no. 15 (April 15, 1933): 1176.

42. Adolf Meyer, "A Science of Man," in *The Commonsense Psychiatry of Adolf Meyer,* ed. Alfred Leif (New York, McGraw-Hill, 1948) p. 539.

43. Stanley Cobb, *Neurology in America,* vol. 2 of *Handbook of Psychiatry,* ed. S. Arieta (New York: Basic Books, 1959), p. 1639.

44. Israel S. Wechsler, *A Textbook of Clinical Neurology* (Philadelphia: W. B. Saunders Co., 1927-1953).

45. Israel S. Wechsler, *The Neuroses* (Philadelphia: W. B. Saunders Co., 1929).

46. Vernon Branham, *Archives of Neurology and Psychiatry* 26, no. 1 (July 1931): 219.

47. "Proceedings of the Nineteenth Congress of the German Neurological Association (1929)," *Archives of Neurology and Psychiatry* 25 (February 1931): 423.

48. Wechsler, *A Textbook of Clinical Neurology,* p. 746.

49. William Graves, "Some Factors Tending Toward Adequate Instruction in Nervous and Mental Diseases," *JAMA* 68, no. 20 (November 1914): 1707.

50. Edward A. Strecker, "Military Psychiatry," in *One Hundred Years of American Psychiatry,* p. 388.

51. Henry Bunker, "Psychiatry as a Specialty," in *One Hundred Years of American Psychiatry,* p. 485.

52. John C. Whitehorn, "Psychiatric Research," in *One Hundred Years of American Psychiatry*, p. 172.

53. Casamajor, "Notes for an Intimate History," p. 604.

54. Cornelius Wholey, "The Menace of Mental Factors in Bodily Diseases," *JAMA* 95, no. 15 (October 11, 1930): 1073.

55. *Medical Education in Brooklyn, The First Hundred Years*, ed. A. Jablons (Brooklyn, N.Y.: State University of New York, Downstate Medical Center, 1960), p. 47.

56. Joseph Globus and Israel Strauss, "Neuro-pathological Cases from Mt. Sinai, May, 1930, Meeting, New York Neurological Society," *Archives of Neurology and Psychiatry* 25, no. 1 (January 1931): 208.

57. Israel Strauss and Joseph H. Globus, "Spongioblastoma Multiforme; A Primary Malignant Form of Brain Neoplasm," *Archives of Neurology and Psychiatry* 14 (August 1925): 139-91.

58. C. Davison, S. P. Goodhart, and W. Needles, "Cerebral Localization in Cerebral Vascular Disease," *Archives of Neurology and Psychiatry* 30 (October 1933): 749.

59. Louis Hausman and Walter Bromberg, "Diabetic Exopthalmic Dysostosis," *Archives of Neurology and Psychiatry* 21 (June 1929): 1402.

60. Arthur Schueller, "Pituitary Dysostosis," *Journal of Nervous and Mental Disease* 64 no. 1 (July 1926): 46.

61. Smith E. Jelliffe, Book reviews, *Journal of Nervous and Mental Disease* 64 no. 3 (September 1926): 261-65.

62. Morris Fishbein, *An Autobiography* (Garden City, N.Y.: Doubleday & Co., 1969), p. 129.

63. Smith E. Jelliffe, "Post-encephalitic Respiratory Disorders," *Journal of Nervous and Mental Disease* 64 no. 1 (July 1926): 29, 157.

64. Smith E. Jelliffe, "Psychologic Components in Post-encephalitic Oculogyric Crises, Contributions to a Genetic Interpretation of Compulsive Phenomena," *Archives of Neurology and Psychiatry* 21 (1929): 491.

65. Lawrence Kubie, Book review, *Psychoanalytic Quarterly* 2 (1933): 622.

66. Sigmund Freud, *New Introductory Lectures* (New York: W. W. Norton, 1933), p. 178.

67. Clarence Oberndorf, *A History of Psychoanalysis in America*, p. 133.

68. Smith E. Jelliffe, "Glimpses of a Freudian Odyssey," *Psychoanalytic Quarterly* 2 (1933): 318.

69. George E. Daniels, "Review of Sketches in Psychomatic Medicine," *Psychoanalytic Quarterly* 10 (1941): 320.

70. Ibid., p. 322.

71. Karl Menninger, "Somatic Correlations With the Unconscious

Repudiation of Femininity in Women," *Journal of Nervous and Mental Disease* 89 no. 4 (April 1939): 514.

72. Karl Menninger, "A Psychiatrist's World: Contribution of Psychoanalysis to American Psychiatry," in *Selected Papers,* ed. Bernard H. Hill (New York: Viking Press, 1959), p. 834.

73. *Archives of Neurology and Psychiatry,* vol. 23, 24, 25, 26 (1927-1931).

74. Bernard Hart, "Psychology and Psychiatry," *Mental Hygiene* 16 (April 1932): 177.

75. Louis Casamajor, "Brain Fever," *JAMA* 149 (August 16, 1952): 1443.

76. Lawson Lowrey, "Treatment of Behavior Problems in Childhood," *Archives of Neurology and Psychiatry* 25 (January 1931): 884.

77. Oswald H. Boltz, "Some Factors which Determine Schizophrenic (Dementia Praecox) Reactions in Males," *Journal of Nervous and Mental Disease* 64 no. 5 (November 1926): 456.

78. Pierce Clark, "A Further Contribution to the Psychology of the Essential Epileptic," *Journal of Nervous and Mental Disease* 63 (May 1923): 575-85.

3

OF STATE HOSPITALS

For the psychiatric neophyte, state hospital service seemed a natural step. During the 1920s some progress had been made in caring for mental patients in institutions. As Adolf Meyer said when he left neuropathology for a broader view of mental illness, "Treatment of the insane must begin before the patient is dead."[1] Indeed, the career of the acknowledged dean of American psychiatry represented a paradigm of this new orientation, the evolution of "living psychiatry." As a neuropathologist at the Eastern State Hospital in Illinois in 1893, organizer of scientific methods at the Worcester State Hospital in 1895, developer of the Pathological Institute in New York in 1903, which was renamed the Psychiatric Institute in 1908, inspiriter of modern psychiatry at the Henry Phipps Psychiatric Clinic in 1913, and author of the *Outline of Psychiatric Examination*, which appeared in 1930, Meyer's career paralelled the evolution of the psychiatric hospital.[2]

For myself, a state hospital experience appeared to be essential at the termination of my neurological residency. I relished the prospect of experiencing the new "living psychiatry" in a state hospital. Before detailing that story, however, it is necessary to outline the interrelation between the mental hygiene movement and institutional psychiatry.

MENTAL HYGIENE IN THE STATE HOSPITAL

Although it was a part of the social reform drive of the early part of this century, the mental health movement was initiated by one man. Clifford Beers's book, *A Mind That Found Itself*, and his vigorous and persistent propaganda to expose the cruelties in asylums became the flag around which progressive psychiatrists rallied.[3] Adolf Meyer had commented on reading Beers's manuscript before its publication, "It looks at last as if we had what we need . . . a man for a cause."[4] The mental hygiene movement, essentially an American idea, eventually spread its message to state hospitals. That the "cause" was initiated by a recovered patient added to its significance. Beers understood this: At the twenty-fifth anniversary meeting of the National Committee for Mental Hygiene in 1934, he reminisced, "After the book was out and I said I was going to start this national and international movement, again my sanity was brought under suspicion . . . seemingly delusions of grandeur." But they were not delusions.

Prominent psychiatrists joined Beers in his wish to befriend the insane and to spread an attitude among the public that mental illness was no more blameworthy than measles. Dr. Frankwood Williams, Dr. Thomas Salmon, and others, working through the National Committee for Mental Hygiene from 1918 onward, agreed with Meyer that the need was "to reach the public" through prevention. The earliest target, aside from gathering sorely needed information about state hospitals throughout the country, was juvenile delinquency. Dr. William Healy had already begun to analyze delinquent children in Chicago's Juvenile Psychopathic Institute. Spurred by this pioneer work, the national committee extended the study of children through fellowships in child guidance centers that were underwritten by the Commonwealth Fund in 1922. Although for years voices had pleaded for the emancipation of children from both the tyranny of the factory and the docility of the "Little Lord Fauntleroy" image, the child guidance movement brought child behavior problems directly under psychiatric scrutiny.[5] Leo Kanner at Johns Hopkins University, a pioneer in child psychiatry, noted that psychiatrists knew little of children's behavior problems until the "beginning of serious, scientific study . . . [to] comprehend and treat personal disorders . . . experienced by young human beings."[6]

The first efforts aimed at educating the public about children's disorders; the second, at preventing mental illness through the treatment of juvenile delinquency and childhood behavior problems.

Defective delinquents, those recognized as unable to control their misbehavior, were considered most important. Inevitably this concern led to mental deficiency in its various forms.[7] While in previous periods, defectives were kept at home, now they were sent to state schools for training. The Hospital Development Commission in New York State already had begun to develop the "travelling clinic: to ferret out disturbed children in the rural regions. . . . Our outpatient clinic in mental hygiene work is a most valuable asset," wrote Sanger Brown in 1919.[8]

The theory of hereditary factors as causes for mental deficiency was still viable at the time. Dr. V. C. Branham, as a member of the New York State system caring for delinquent defectives at the Woodbourne Institution, echoed this viewpoint in 1926: "The hereditary and enviromental background of these men is startlingly unsound. . . . Our study vindicates the theory that the defective delinquent . . . is to be segregated for special study and care."[9] Emphasis on childhood problems even extended to outside the hospital.[10] Books, written by educators and psychiatrists and aimed at preventing behavior problems in children at home, appeared in great numbers. Works like Richardson's *Re-Building the Child*, Galloway's *Parenthood and the Character Training of the Child,* Dr. Douglas Thom's *Mental Health of the Child,* were expected to prevent behavior disturbances in clinics and hospitals by educating the public.[11]

The social worker, whose ministrations started with Mary Potter Meyer's visits to patients' homes in New York's Harlem early in the century, came into existence as a means of bringing mental health to citizens. At the behest of her husband, Dr. Adolf Meyer, then at the Pathological Institute on Ward's Island in New York, she interviewed the parents and neighbors of patients, amassing information about the environment, social pressures, and personality types, which preceded the patient's hospitalization. Mary Potter Meyer's visits and her subsequent reports to the doctor eventually blossomed into the field of psychiatric social work.[12] In a short time, Dr. Meyer said that "her work became absolutely indispensable."[13]

By 1919 the goals of this "indispensable worker" were firmly set. Lectures and courses in psychiatric social work were established at Smith College in Northhampton, Massachusetts, and Simmons College in Boston. Such leaders in the child guidance movement as E. E. Southard, Mary Jarrett, chief social worker at the Boston Psychopathic Hospital, and Lawson Lowrey became the new idols for an early generation of trained social workers.[14] As they entered the state hospital system in New York in 1906 and Massachusetts in 1919, they became the shock troops used in interpreting mental illness to patients' relatives. Edith Spaulding best enunciated their aim: "The field of psychiatric social work . . . through understanding the true interpretation of mental symptoms, is . . . able to spread in the community an attitude encouraging treatment in early stages."[15] Their efforts, joined with psychiatrists, psychologists, pediatricians, and others, resulted in the creation of the Orthopsychiatric Association, which was organized in 1924. From this amalgam sprang the notion of a treatment "team."[16]

The momentum initiated by Orthopsychiatric Association spread to other preventive psychiatric efforts. Industry, schools, psychopathic hospitals, courts, and state hospitals reacted positively to mental hygiene principles.[17] Moreover, authoritative and enjoyable books, like Karl M. Menninger's *The Human Mind,* informed the reading public.[18] Menninger's book, a Literary Guild selection in 1930, made the best-seller list. "In many minds," a biographer of the Menninger family noted, "the Menninger name and psychiatry became indivisible."[19] By the 1930s the meaning of mental health had become unmistakably imprinted on the subliminal American mind. As the movement gained adherents, it developed a kind of ebullience, evidenced in a euphoric comment by the *Mental Hygiene* journal in 1928:

Mental Hygiene presents wide aspects. . . . [It] has a message also for those who consider themselves normal, for by its aims, the man who is fifty per cent efficient can make himself seventy per cent; the man seventy percent, perhaps eighty percent; and so on.[20]

Still, the ardor for the total mental benefit of mankind had its critics. Israel Wechsler, a neurologist, in an article for the *Journal of the American Medical Association* in 1930 cast a jaundiced eye on "enthusiastic mental hygienists [who] tell us that it is concerned with prevention of mental deficiency, criminality, the psychoneuroses, the psychoses, antisocial traits, family unhappiness, divorce, alcoholism, sexual perversion, epilepsy, and other such simple matters. . . . How do we know?"[21] And in a less cynical vein, Professor Charles Emerson wrote: "The Mental Hygiene movement has proven interesting to the public; very gratifying but also dangerous. . . . Psychiatrists have a duty to warn the public regarding new vistas and . . . alluring possibilities . . . [that] may not be justified."[22]

Growth of State Hospitals

In spite of carping criticisms, which were not without merit, the publicity arising from the mental hygiene movement stimulated the expansion of state hospital patient populations. An editorial in a New York newspaper in 1927, as reported in the *Psychiatric Quarterly*, stated:

It is no doubt true that because of newspaper publicity the State Hospitals for the care and treatment of the mentally ill have become widely and more favorably known among the people of the State . . . [giving an] increase in confidence. . . . The mild cases formerly treated at home are now being sent to institutions . . . [for] better than average care.[23]

Statisticians in the Department of Mental Hygiene in New York diligently studied this increase in hospital admissions. Dr. Horatio Pollack found that patients "on the books" had doubled between 1924 and 1928.[24] When he sought to estimate the future population of state hospitals, he remarked that preventive methods were "gaining ground but difficulties abounded." The present methods, Pollack reminded his readers, were "established in a pre-mental hygiene age." According to Pollack, what was needed "as the new science of mental hygiene develops are new systems of human relationships, new habits, new customs, new standards and ideals. . . . In the meantime . . . we need to be equipped to receive many thousand mental patients . . . before the mental hygiene millenium arrives." New York State, at least, felt the pressure and responded by floating a $50 million bond in 1924 for erecting new hospitals and refurbishing old ones. Governor

Alfred E. Smith enthusiastically agreed. Three years later at the cornerstone laying for the Psychiatric Institute near where the Columbia Medical Center was raising its impressive head on Washington Heights, he remarked, "If these patients are to increase at the rate of nearly 2,000 a year, that means a new hospital every two years."[25]

Aside from the possibilities of successful treatment, which the public was beginning to perceive, two influences within the profession itself were responsible for increases in hospital patient population: the prompting of Meyerian teaching, and the entrance of dynamic thinking in the psychiatrists' armamentarium. The first influence was contiguous to, and partly arose out of, mental hygiene as a social reform drive. To understand the effect that Meyer exerted from 1910 to 1930, it must be remembered that state hospital and asylum physicians had just mastered Kraepelin's diagnostic system, which had brought order out of the chaotic bundle of symptoms they faced in their patients. The monumental work of Eugen Bleuler in analyzing and renaming dementia praecox, his differentiation of primary and secondary (principal and accessory) symptoms of schizophrenia, shed light on what appeared to be an inexplicable mass of peculiar behavior and utterances.[26] "Amentias, paranoid states, monomanias, atypical melancholias" all fell into place under the rubric of schizophrenia. As Bleuler stated, "After paresis was excluded from among the 'functional psychoses' and other organic forms followed of themselves, for seventy years theoretical psychiatry stood entirely helpless before the chaos of the most frequent mental diseases."[27] Bleuler's concepts of a unitary disease, schizophrenia in its four types, cleared the air. Diagnosis and prognosis could be made with assurance. Dr. Brill told me several years later how he had solved a perplexing case brought to him by Dr. Tilney, a professor of neurology, after weeks of unavailing neurological and medical tests at Columbia Medical Center. "A brief history and one look told me it was schizophrenia." He added with a wink, "We didn't need all those tests."

In spite of this advance in understanding, therapeutic measures for chronic psychoses eluded physicians. Bleuler's conclusion in his chapter on schizophrenia sounded fatal: "Schizophrenics are not to be treated at all." Yet for American psychiatrists, mental hygiene's message of hope, especially for prevention, and Meyer's commonsense attitude combined to lighten the pervasive dead-endedness with which chronic psychotics were viewed. Meyer never tired of saying to his psychiatric listeners, "We must get away from the idea that one examines only for some all-inclusive asylum disease like dementia praecox and manic-depressive insanity and paresis."[28] He proved time and again that there was a way to tease out the factors that underlay the psychosis, that psychiatrists were dealing with a plastic, not yet concrete, mode of thinking and behavior in their patients: "One examines primarily for the range of personal capacity . . . in any plan for treatment; that is, assets as shown in plain life problems and successes and failures."[29]

THE MANHATTAN STATE HOSPITAL

After a survey of progressive state hospitals, Iowa Psycho-pathic Hospital and Foxboro State Hospital in Massachusetts at which William Malamud was superintendent and David Roths-child was clinical director, I chose Manhattan State Hospital. It lay on Ward's Island and was equidistant from Harlem's Little Italy to the west and the nondescript shores of Queens Borough on the east. Serene and independent, the island, a largish piece of land that spliced the East River before it divided between the Harlem River and its entrance into Long Island Sound on its northern course, was one of an irregular chain of islands that graced the river. It and the hospital buildings provided an air that could be transformed into a Currier and Ives print of Olde Gotham. The hospital itself covered the body of the island, uncon-cerned with the tumult of Manhattan and its skyscrapers that looked down on it as a country cousin.

Manhattan State Hospital seemed a propitious choice. Some of New York's leading dynamic psychiatrists—Adolph Stern, A. A. Brill, Clarence Oberndorf, Monroe Meyer, and August Hoch—had trained there and at Central Islip State Hospital. I approached the post of assistant physician with an exhilaration that was soon tempered by reality.

The main buildings were a replica of the model planned by Dr. Kirkbride between 1850 and 1880, which was itself an advance over earlier structures.[30] The administration building with its rolltop desks and massive wooden files reflected the period. The buildings that housed the patients were of a single plan: spacious, high-ceilinged main halls that emptied into individual rooms and dormitories, a nurses' station, and a physician's office. Along the walls in the main hall stood a row of straight-backed chairs on which patients sat for hours gazing at a few simple homespun pictures on the walls of bucolic scenes of plates of game or fruit lying in lifeless quietude. A few smaller rooms for disturbed patients boasted heavier chairs on which deteriorated patients were bound, some with diapers because of their loss of sphincter control. The "back wards" occupied a series of solid, red-bricked buildings, that appeared more antiquated as one receded from the administration building. The grounds were well cared for; a modern reception unit, an auditorium, and gardens graced the center of the island. But the cheerfulness of the environs did not penetrate the wards, which were filled with gesticulating, restless, or apathetic patients in contrast to the ward for tuberculosis patients and the infirmary, which presented a medical atmosphere.

The staff was headed by Dr. Floyd Haviland, of whom Dr. Clarence Cheney wrote in 1930, "Dr. Haviland . . . was enthusiastic and receptive towards progressive ideas, looking toward the welfare of mental patients."[31] Between 1927 and 1928 Haviland had been president of the New York Society for Clinical Psychiatry, and he had struggled to change the old order. He hired a group of young psychiatrists apparently to act as stimuli to the "old-timers," those veterans of state hospital service. Of these, Oberndorf, out of his early experience, wrote: "The older physicians . . . habituated to the routine of custodial care . . . growled and chaffed . . . at the time-consuming new methods." They offered quips "about Fraud and Junk (Freud and Jung) . . . but could not openly defy what their leaders approved."[32] Even earlier, A. A. Brill had noted their resistance to the careful note-taking methods that Meyer introduced at the Pathological Institute. In place of Meyer's carefully documented observation notes, the older physicians had written of patients: "Dull, stupid, demented."

While the younger doctors, Brill noted, followed the examination outline "implicitly," the veterans snorted, "Why write so many notes and waste so much time?"[33] One of the older physicians pensively confided to me of the "millions of words" he had written in the ledger books that served as permanent records in the old days.

A main duty of the hospital physician was to control disturbed patients. Dr. Folsom, assistant superintendent, counseled new physicians, "Remember, the patients are afraid of you. . . . Keep the keys in your mitt at all times." One sensed the ancient fear of the insane in the attitudes of older physicians. The infusion of implied hope by the newer psychiatrists, bolstered by their determination to ferret out hidden complexes, was generally greeted as an innovation without substance. A century of discarded innovations in the care of the insane had hardened into an appreciation of the adage, "Once insane, always insane." It was not that the older men did not recognize psychopathology but that delusions and neologisms had long since lost their meaning and allure. One veteran confided in me his perplexity: "Some patients look like dementia praecox for three days, then like manic-depressives for three days."

After an initial orientation period in the modern reception building, I was assigned to a vast structure, which was fronted by the legend INEBRIATE ASYLUM, 1854, to care for the 400 chronic patients therein. My wife and I were assigned an apartment in this building under the care of a chronic patient who cleaned the rooms and left little symbolic mementos for the "new patients." A spinster-lady, the then accepted designation for unmarried women, Miss McDonald relished her job, which she believed included protecting my wife and me from the evil machinations of the Black Hand. After each morning's housework, she left counter-charms on the bureau to ward off any designs the Black Hand gangs "who were everywhere" might have on her charges. The charms consisted of a paper band formed into a plinth, which was surrounded by a black ribbon at the base. The symbolism of Miss McDonald's charms could, and were, interpreted freely.

My clinical assignment included evaluating the 400 patients domiciled in the erstwhile inebriate asylum, some of whom had not been seen by a psychiatrist for years. It proved to be a lonely but fascinating task as I interviewed and annotated four or five each day. The senior physician, under whose aegis I worked, showed little interest in the psychopathology I dredged up in the older cases. Dr. K., a genial Vermonter who accepted his job as a sinecure against a small practice in town, arrived on the ward at 9:30 A.M., signed a few orders for the day, engaged in small talk with the nurses, left for lunch, and returned around 2:00 P.M. for more conversation until the day ended for him at 4:00 P.M.

Routine on the back wards was drab, hopeless, eternal. The Slough of Despond that characterized the chronic wards received an occasional ray of light through the kindnesses of the attendants. These men and women, chiefly recent Irish immigrants with brogues as thick as a London fog, maintained a warm regard for their charges. Their friendliness without condescension or affectation contained a trace of the monastic tradition of centuries ago, when the religious treated the "frenzied" with kindness and paternalism. Among the female attendants, it took the form of bestowing bits of finery on patients they fancied; the male attendants tried to inspirit young males with "spunk," the equivalent of today's "macho." Occasionally entertainment was offered in the auditorium, and the patients dutifully listened. Once, my wife, an interpretative dancer, performed a Nautch dance in native costume adorned with bells; the dramatic effect stimulated an epileptic in the audience to "throw a fit," as the attendants explained. The Christmas season evoked a flurry of decoration—wreaths of holly and religious picture—that were stripped away on the second day of January to reveal even emptier wards by contrast.

An unstructured recreation program for the men of the inebriate asylum included an informal handball game against a stout brick wall near the building where attendants and patients played on cold winter afternoons. Often Samuel Atkin, our fellow tenant, and I joined the game. Mixing with patients was a frowned upon activity, but Atkin and I enjoyed the camaraderie in a game where social-psychological disparities were leveled, where the sane and insane concentrated only on the thwack of a hard rubber ball against a brick wall. With no one realizing it, the daily doctor-patient game served as a kind of wordless group therapy.

In the hospital, the chief nurse, and my handball partner, Pat
Browne worked with the same sense of undefined camaraderie.
One of our duties was the daily tube-feeding of catatonic patients
who refused to eat. Each afternoon, with the precision of a well-
trained drill master, Browne lined up the patients in bed, slipped
the rubber tubes deftly into the nostrils, while I checked the
improbability of their entering the larynx, and produced the
solution of milk, eggs, and sugar, which I poured into the funnel.
The catatonic patients, as if sensing the humanity of Browne's
ministrations, lay supine, bodies rigid, but eyes alert, watching
the procedure with expressions of faint gratitude. Within half an
hour, Pat Browne and I had given fifteen to eighteen patients
their liquid meals.

Other ward buildings presented the same dismal atmosphere of
chronicity. One of the older structures housed several dungeons
in the basement that reminded one of the scene that greeted
Phillipe Pinel a century and a half ago at the Bicêtre in Paris,
although they had not been used for decades. The ambience
of asylum days lingered on in the pharmacy, which was appro-
priately located in the basement. Here the chief pharmacist,
surrounded by vials, funnels, huge bottles, and scales, earnestly
poured gallons of rhubarb and soda, milk of magnesia, and nux
vomica into bottles for distribution to the wards. The choice of
antipsychotic medications was limited—Luminal for epileptics,
morphine and hyoscine for disturbed patients, bromides for
nervous tension. The pharmacist, a small intense man with a
Teutonic accent and corresponding *Sitzfleisch*, presided patiently
and diligently over his aromatic stock like a gnome in the underworld. He surfaced only for lunch, worried aloud about shipments
of drugs that invariably arrived late, ate a hasty meal, and slipped
off to the unsung theme of the *Nibelungenlied*.

The Staff

The lugubrious picture of the back wards was more than com-
pensated for by the staff conferences. Run by Dr. Lonergan, the
clinical director, a wiry Irishman with an underslung wit and the
perpetual half smile of a leprechaun, the discussions turned chiefly

on Kraepelinian, sometimes Bleulerian, diagnoses. The staff, which was a mixture of neophytes and veterans, included Remé Breguét, the scion of an honored Swiss family of horological fame, George Swetlow, a New York innovative neurosurgeon, two genial Texans who were chiefly stirred by the delights New York City afforded, several young Canadians from the Maritime Provinces, an exchange student from Westphalia, Germany, a sober, nonexpressive expatriate from Russia, and a French physician from Quebec who was bewildered by references to such foreign notions as "libido," "symbolism," and "transference." The younger group of native New Yorkers, who were bent on reading dynamic meaning into the patient's symptoms and utterances, were balanced by two older veterans of state service who were resigned to the eternal task of differentiating manic from excited paranoid patients.

The problems confronting the staff rarely extended beyond mere diagnoses. Occasionally the bleak therapeutic picture was relieved by the spontaneous recovery of a catatonic patient. Dr. Bloomfield, a psychiatrist in charge of one of the chronic wards, reported such a recovery in which the patient suddenly came out of her stupor and said "I'm all right" after thirteen years in the hospital. The story appeared on the front page of the *New York Times,* while the staff argued about the cause of this astonishing denouement. In fact, spontaneous recovery of catatonic patients occurred in other New York hospitals fairly frequently. James May in a thorough study, entitled *The Dementia Praecox-Schizophrenia Problem,* declared that those schizophrenics who recovered were actually cases of psychopathic personality, mental deficiency, traumatic conditions, or involutional states, who "do not deteriorate . . . [and have] episodic illnesses . . . [which] undoubtedly explains the recovery rate."[34] Others in the state hospital service reported recoveries of schizophrenics. For example, in 1930, 35 out of 592 admissions were reported as recovered, indicating that the dictum "dementia praecox cases cannot recover . . . [to be] too rigid adherence to this dogma."[35] Another psychiatrist, C. H. Bellinger at the Brooklyn State Hospital, reported one-quarter of his group of catatonic patients could "adjust to extramural life" with the aid of social service follow-up, parole contacts

in their home environment, and occupational therapy.[36] Some of
the hopelessness was beginning to fade.

SCIENCE AND PSYCHIATRY

The activities in the Psychiatric Institute, housed on the less
antiquated end of Ward's Island, were even more promising. The
institute had functioned as a springboard for Adolf Meyer's epoch-
making improvements in state hospital practice. Meyer had
stimulated the formation of a pathological laboratory at the
institute, and Dr. Dunlap, the pathologist, had studied hundreds
of brains of deceased dementia praecox cases in a vain search for
some telltale, neuropathologic lesion of this dread disease. Satisfied with the nonproductiveness of neuropathology in the schizophrenic conundrum, Meyer recommended studying everything
pertinent to the life of the patient. "Mind cannot be found in the
brain," he concluded, "it must be found in the record."[37] He was
impatient with those trying to "translate things into brain mythology." This new approach to dementia praecox cases constituted his commonsense attitude. "It is far from conceivable,"
he wrote, "that [dementia praecox] . . . was due to invented
poisons or things back of it all." From this viewpoint, he developed
his "distributive analysis," a treatment which made "unavoidable
difficulties acceptable to the patient . . . assigned a share in
factors in the patient's troubles . . . desensitized the sore points
showing how these factors could be managed . . . prepared the
patient to use his or her own resources."[38]

Meyer's therapeutic technique stood in contrast to that of the
analysts. His bedside manner, which I observed on a visit to the
Phipps Institute, was unobtrusive, his speech subdued, and his
approach reminiscent of a minister visiting the sick. There may
have been a dignified consolation in his style, but it hid his
careful observations. His patience and attentiveness to the subject
in hand caused Paul Schilder to remark after a day-long meeting
of the American Psychiatric Association at which Meyer presided,
"Meyer is admirable."

When George Kirby, professor of psychiatry at Columbia
University, succeeded to Meyer's position, the latter's influence

was perceptible. Kirby added a somatic approach, especially the new von Jauregg malaria treatment for general paralysis, which was imported from Vienna. This breakthrough in the treatment of an obdurate disease earned Wagner von Jauregg the Nobel Prize for medicine in 1927. The malaria strain was carried to Ward's Island to a ward full of paretic patients, and the subsequent sharp fever rises, controlled by quinine, seemed to stem their extravagant delusions and disorganized thinking.[39]

Under Kirby's leadership, research in many phases of clinical psychiatry continued. After successes with malaria inoculation in which raised body temperature presumably accounted for improvement, a heat cabinet was developed with the hope of more precisely controlling temperature increases.[40] Another area of psychobiologic research dealt with Henry Cotton's focal infection theory as the cause of mental disease. At the New Jersey State Hospital in Trenton, Cotton had acted on his notion that the functional mental illnesses arose "from circulating toxins originating in foci of infection."[41] The removal of teeth, tonsils, gall bladder, prostates, uterine cervices, colons, and sinuses in the interest of curing mental diseases appeared to be a breakthrough. Although the focal infection theory spread as a boon to mental patients glowing hopes for curing schizophrenia and other diseases faded abruptly. At the Psychiatric Institute, Nicholas Kopeloff, a research bacteriologist, proved after a carefully controlled study that Cotton's theory was illusory.[42] The miracle cure subsided within a few years. In 1928 Sanger Brown described the focal infection theory as "a cure-all . . . attractive to the laity," and went on to say, "but that does not make it scientifically sound."[43]

Still the quest for somatic treatment for psychotic persons continued: Prolonged narcosis with barbituates, stimulation by strychnine, hormone preparations, and oxygen injections were tried.[44] Epilepsy among other chronic conditions did not yield to bromide medications. At Manhattan State Hospital, John Notkin worked endlessly to control the daily seizures in a ward full of idiopathic epileptics, some of whom were mentally deteriorated after years of major seizures. Without the benefit of the undiscovered electroencephalograph, Notkin and Professor Pike, a neurophysiologist at Columbia, experimented diligently to find a cause for this obdurate condition.[45]

Besides the convulsive state other organic problems begged for attention at the hospital. Our neurological consultant, Samuel Burchell of the New York Neurologic Institute, made weekly visits to examine the organic cases that Atkin and I gathered from among the apparent hulks in the back wards. Among these were bizarre sequellae of the encephalitis epidemics of 1920 to 1924. One such was a thirteen-year-old boy whose respiratory tics, peculiar compulsive rotary movement, and oculogyric crises combined with behavior disturbances had caused his commitment to the state hospital. The flood of tics, snorting speech, and respiratory grunts, which were caused by the pathologic changes in his basal ganglia, interfered with an otherwise not abnormal mentality. The patient's clinical picture presented a fascinating *Grenzgebiete* (borderline) between neurology and psychiatry. The oculogyric tic particularly reminded one of Jelliffe's analysis of oculogyric crises among catatonics as symbolic expressions of castration. At several academy meetings and in his writings, Jelliffe had demonstrated a common symptomatology among chronic encephalitis and catatonics in which release of cerebral inhibition and psychological conflicts eventuated in similar clinical pictures. His study of *Postencephalitic Respiratory Disorders,* for example, demonstrated on analysis the "repetition compulsion" found among compulsive neurotics.[46]

Pursuing the chronic encephalitis problem, I found 135 cases admitted for bizarre movement disturbances and tics who were regarded as catatonic schizophrenics. Most were from the files; a few were currently on the back wards. Following an analysis of these cases, which was published in the *Psychiatric Quarterly* under the title "Mental State in Chronic Encephalitis,"[47] two were selected for presentation at an Academy of Medicine meeting.[48] In this · presentation I emphasized the remarkable correspondence between functional mental disease and organic conditions. Besides the boy with the respiratory tics and rotary body movements, an adult exhibiting narcolepsy and cataplexy after an acute encephalitic infection was demonstrated.

The Leading Edge of Psychiatry

In addition to the work with malarial treatment of paresis, the major thrust of research at the Psychiatric Institute on Ward's

Island dealt with dynamic interpretations of psychotic symptoms, which until then had been nominated as "bizarre" and hence unanalyzable. Thus, Theodore Robie analyzed the Oedipus and homosexual complexes in schizophrenic patients; Leland Hinsie studied symbolism in neurotic cases; and C. S. Wolff scrutinized catatonic behavior in dementia praecox patients.[49] The monthly meetings at the institute began to demonstrate the encroachment of psychoanalysis. For example, Dorian Feigenbaum, the future editor of the *Psychoanalytic Quarterly,* gave a detailed report on his analysis of a paranoid psychotic, a condition that until 1930 had been considered impervious to psychological interpretation. Indeed by 1933, William A. White was able to say "[What] psychoanalysis did for psychiatry was to open the door to the understanding of patients which strangely had been heretofore closed. . . . Patient's remarks were [considered to be] of no significance because they were crazy or incoherent."[50] Frankwood Williams went further: writing in the first issue of the *Psychoanalytic Quarterly* in 1932, he suggested that although "among sympathetic psychiatrists who have no firsthand knowledge of psychoanalysis, it has become the custom to speak of psychoanalysis with enthusiasm . . . but only as a special technique for specific illness."[51] The leading edge of psychiatric research, he wrote, should go to the very "motivation of human conduct."

The intriguing area of schizophrenic treatment possibilities lay at the center of discussion. Manfred Bleuler, the son of Eugen Bleuler, lectured at Bloomingdale Hospital in 1930 on the ineffectiveness of treatment methods. He declared, "nothing found to date influences the primary process," which his father had enucleated from the schizophrenic process, and added that "apparent cures are spontaneous remissions" and that psychoanalysis exerted "no direct effect on schizophrenic patients."[52] In spite of this fiat from Zurich, American psychiatrists continued to experiment with dynamic treatment. Franz Alexander averred that "simple and uncritical imitation of treatment for neurosis" could not be applied to schizophrenics.[53] Bernard Glueck in his private sanitarium in Ossining, New York, urged "less rigidity," and Frieda Fromm-Reichmann at Shepard and Enoch Pratt in Maryland experimented with variations in analytic technique as did Harry Stack Sullivan.[54]

Under the stimulus of these innovations the dread final stage of schizophrenic deterioration became less frightening. Psychodynamic investigations led the way and made psychoanalysis more and more attractive to younger members of the hospital staff. Much of our conversations away from the wards dealt with dream interpretation, symbolisms, and defenses in our own lives and that of our patients. When one of the older staff members died of pneumonia, a drawer full of razor blades found in his quarters occasioned an interpretation of fetishism. Since the deceased was a bachelor, the conclusion of latent homosexuality seemed inevitable. In this context Samuel Atkin, already embarked on his psychoanalytical training, urged me to undertake a didactic analysis with his analyst, Abram Kardiner. Atkin's enthusiasm for the horizon that opened before him was persuasive.

The reasons for plunging into the swelling tide of psychoanalytical training were more than academic. Unless the young psychiatrist wished to remain in state institutional service, analysis offered the best chance for a better-than-average income. As a status symbol, it could not be excelled. Once one had assimilated the concept and derivatives of unconscious mentation, he joined a coterie of physicians who, at least in their own estimation, rose above grubby medical siblings who probed the flesh and studied the detritus of suffering patients. We felt there was something noble and elevating in dealing with symbols, lofty concepts, and higher abstractions. Besides the allure of esoteric language about neurotic patients, the freedom to investigate sexual matters cast a special glamour over the new profession; the opportunity to explore the hitherto muted sexual experience of men and (especially) women was now clothed in scientific respectablity.

Karl Menninger once alluded to the seductive quality of psychosexual investigations in discussing these "obstreperous and preposterous Freudians," who at an American Psychiatric Association meeting in the early 1920s, "under the impact of Brill, popped up with psychoanalytic interpretation." Shocked at the familiarity with esoterica displayed by the analysts, the young Karl, who was not yet indoctrinated, thought: "What was the world coming to when New Yorkers come to a dignified meeting and talk about sex . . . and such sex!"[55]

One other concern, though not voiced openly, strongly influenced young, especially Jewish, psychiatrists to become analysts:
namely, the Talmudic preoccupation with convoluted thinking and
intricate suppositions. The kind of cerebration that psychoanalysis
demanded, resting in large part on analogy, metaphor, and
intuition, was far different and hence more intriguing than that
required in medicine proper. In the idiom of the day it was a
"natural" for the intellectual physician. As John Burnham has
pointed out, the intelligentsia had early espoused psychoanalysis,
and "psychoanalysis continued for many decades to play the
avant-garde role in substantial portions of American culture."[56]
More specifically, Burnham stated, "The new sponsors of psychoanalysis were members of the WASP-Jewish elite who came to
dominate American cultural institutions from the 1930s to the
1960s.[57]

In spite of this historical truth, some of us remained on the
periphery of analytic candidacy, for reasons both rational and
obscure. At the same time, the pressures to undergo analysis
were oblique but strong. Besides sociocultural factors, economic
ones played a part. Paul Roazen in his *Freud and His Followers*
makes a point rarely discussed in the literature: "By 1924 psychoanalysis was becoming a successful method of making a living. The
economic factors in the history of psychoanalysis can easily be
overlooked."[58] Speaking of psychoanalysis and medical education,
Allen Gregg, a prominent psychiatrist and mental hygienist,
assumed the prosperity of analysis when he asked, "[Can] psychoanalysis now face the task of surviving prosperity in the form of
admission to academic status?"[59] For myself, financial considerations outweighed theoretical ones in 1929. I had a hospital income
of $1,800 per year that excluded subsistence and included a newly
arrived daughter. In any case, if I had emotional problems—
Ferenczi and Rank had written, "Behind every desire for a so-called
didactic analysis lies the more or less urgent need for an actual
analysis"—I concluded they were egosyntonic.[60]

Finally, there were other factors disfavoring entrance into the
celestial city. It became obvious that the two fields of psychiatry
and neurology were drifting apart. Neurologists argued about
localization of lesions, microscopic findings, and differential

diagnosis; psychiatrists discussed nebulous concepts like the ego, id, and superego. An air of contention surrounded psycho-analytical activity, whereas neurology was bathed in scholarly ambience. The cleavages between the Freudians, Jungians, Rankians, and Adlerians, not to mention the claims of Stekelians (Stekel urged a shortening of the analytic process), almost amounted to religious wars.

Despite this internecine warfare, both bewildering and amusing to the neophyte, I felt there was more to psychiatry than could be observed in a state hospital. I wished to see, for example, the vast array of acute problems facing neurologists and psychiatrists in active practice. An acute psychiatric service in a university hospital seemed desirable. In 1930 the psychiatric division of Bellevue Hospital in conjunction with New York University had increased its staff in response to a larger patient load. I applied for the position of junior psychiatrist, was accepted, and thereby entered a new psychiatric world.

NOTES

1. Adolf Meyer, *Collected Works,* ed. Eunice Winters (Baltimore, Md.: Johns Hopkins Press, 1951), pp. 63, 78, 100.

2. Adolf Meyer, *The Commonsense Psychiatry of Dr. Adolf Meyer,* ed. Alfred Lief (New York: McGraw-Hill, 1948).

3. Clifford Beers, *A Mind that Found Itself, An Autobiography* (Garden City, N.Y.: Doubleday, Doran and Co., 1937).

4. Meyer, *Commonsense Psychiatry,* p. 280.

5. Ellen Key, *The Century of the Child,* trans. M. Franzos, (New York: G. P. Putnam, 1909).

6. Leo Kanner, *Child Psychiatry,* 3d ed. (Springfield, Ill.: Charles C. Thomas, 1957), p. 9.

7. George J. Veith, "Training the Idiot and Imbecile," *Psychiatric Quarterly* 1 (1927): 70.

8. Sanger Brown II, "The Care of Mental Defectives in New York State," *Psychiatric Quarterly* 1 (1927): 146.

9. V. C. Branham, "Notes on the Classification of Defective Delinquents," *Journal of Criminal Law and Criminology* 27, no. 22 (August 1926).

10. Marion Kenworthy, "Extra-medical Services in the Management of

Misconduct Problems in Children," *Mental Hygiene* 5, no. 4 (October 1921): 724.

11. See Frank H. Richardson, *Re-Building of the Child* (Cambridge, Mass.: Harvard University Press, 1928); Thomas W. Galloway, *Parenthood and the Character Training of the Child* (New York: Methodist Book Concern, 1927); and Douglas A. Thom. *Mental Health of the Child* (Cambridge, Mass.: Harvard University Press, 1928).

12. Meyer, *The Commonsense Psychiatry*, p. 149.

13. Ibid.

14. Note, *Mental Hygiene* 3, no. 1 (January 1919): 121.

15. Edith Spaulding, "Training the Psychiatric Social Worker," *Mental Hygiene* 3, no. 1 (January 1919): 420.

16. Announcement, *Mental Hygiene* 10 no. 3 (July 1926): 664.

17. See Macfie Campbell, "Mental Hygiene in Industry," *Mental Hygiene* 5 no. 8 (July 1921): 468; Boyd Fisher, "Has Mental Hygiene a Practical Use in Industry?" *Mental Hygiene* 5, no. 8 (July 1921): 479; Walter L. Treadway, "The Place of Mental Hygiene in the Schools," *American Journal of Public Health* 13 (November 1923): 928; Frankwood Williams, "The Importance of Social Relationships in the Development of the Personality and Character of the Adolescent," *Mental Hygiene* 14 no. 4 (October 1930): 901; Macfie Campbell, "The Work of the Psychopathic Hospital," *Mental Hygiene* 14, no. 4 (October 1930): 883; Note, *Mental Hygiene* 14, no. 4 (October 1930): 499; and Horatio Pollack, "Personnel Relations in the State Hospital," *Mental Hygiene* 6, no. 3 (July 1922): 592.

18. Karl Menninger, *The Human Mind* (New York: Alfred A. Knopf, 1930).

19. Winslow Walker, *The Menninger Story* (Garden City, N.Y.: Doubleday & Co., 1956), p. 207.

20. Editorial, *Mental Hygiene* 12 (1928).

21. Israel S. Wechsler, "The Legend of Prevention of Mental Disease," *Journal of the American Medical Association* (hereafter *JAMA*) 95 (July 5, 1930): 24.

22. Charles P. Emerson, "Mental Hygiene: Wise and Unwise Investments," *Mental Hygiene* 10, no. 3 (July 1926): 449.

23. Editorial reprinted in *Psychiatric Quarterly* 1 (1927): 558.

24. Horatio Pollack, "Increase in Patients in Civil State Hospitals of New York," *Psychiatric Quarterly* 2 (1938): 214.

25. Note, *Psychiatric Quarterly* 2 (1938): 538.

26. Eugen Bleuler, *Textbook of Psychiatry*, trans. A. A. Brill (New York: Macmillan Co., 1924), p. 54.

27. Ibid., p. 372.
28. Adolf Meyer, "Training the Doctors," in *The Commonsense Psychiatry of Dr. Adolf Meyer,* p. 572.
29. Ibid., p. 399.
30. Samuel W. Hamilton, "American Mental Hospitals," in *One Hundred Years of American Psychiatry,* ed. J. K. Hall (New York: Columbia University Press, 1944), p. 95.
31. Clarence C. Cheney, Floyd Haviland Obituary, *Mental Hygiene* 14, no. 1 (January 1930), p. 161.
32. Clarence Oberndorf, *A History of Psychoanalysis in America* (New York: Grune & Stratton, 1953), p. 103.
33. A. A. Brill, "The Role of Psychoanalysis in the Prevention of Mental and Nervous Diseases," *Psychiatric Quarterly* 2 (1928): 289.
34. James V. May, "The Dementia-Schizophrenia Problem," *Psychiatric Quarterly* 6 (1932): 40.
35. H. L. Levin, "Recovery in Dementia Praecox," *Psychiatric Quarterly* 5 (1931): 476.
36. C. H. Bellinger, "Prognosis in Schizophrenia—Catatonic Form," *Psychiatric Quarterly* 6 (1932): 474.
37. Adolf Meyer, "A Science of Man," in *The Commonsense Psychiatry of Dr. Adolf Meyer,* p. 537 et seq.
38. Wendell Muncie, *Psychobiology and Psychiatry,* 2d ed. (St. Louis: C. V. Mosby, 1948), p. 522.
39. Henry A. Bunker and George H. Kirby, "Treatment of General Paralysis by Inoculation with Malaria," *JAMA* 84, no. 8 (February 21, 1925): 563.
40. Leland E. Hinsie and Charles H. Carpenter, "Radio-thermic Treatment of General Paralysis," *Psychiatric Quarterly,* 5 (1931): 215.
41. Henry A. Cotton, "The Etiology and Treatment of the So-called Functional Psychoses: Summary of Results Based on Experience of Four Years," *American Journal of Psychiatry* 2 (October 1922): 157.
42. N. Kopeloff and C. Cheney, "Studies in Focal Infections: Its Presence and Elimination in the Functional Psychoses," *American Journal of Psychiatry* 2 (October 1922): 139.
43. Sanger Brown, "Specialism Within the Field of Psychiatry," *Pschiatric Quarterly* 2 (1928): 9.
44. See Harold Palmer and Alfred Paine, "Prolonged Narcosis as Therapy in the Psychoses," *American Journal of Psychiatry* 12 (July 1932): 143; Leland E. Hinsie and Sigfried Katz, "Treatment of Manic Depressive Psychosis: A Survey of the Literature," *American Journal of Psychiatry* 11 (July 1931) 131; Karl M. Bowman and Lauretta Bender,

"The Treatment of Involutional Melancholia with Ovarian Hormone," *American Journal of Psychiatry* 12 (March 1932): 867; and John Notkin, William Greeff, F. H. Pike, and J. A. Killian, "Changes in the Clincial Signs and Laboratory Findings in Various Types of Psychoses Under the Influence of Subcutaneous Administration of Oxygen," *American Journal of Psychiatry* 12 (May 1933): 1271.

45. John Notkin, "Chloride-Bromide Treatment in Epilepsy," *Archives of Neurology and Psychiatry* 21 (January 1929): 165. There are also many papers in the *American Journal of Psychiatry,* 1928 to 1933.

46. Smith E. Jelliffe, *Post-Encephalitic Respiratory Disorders,* Nervous and Mental Disease Monograph Series, no. 45 (Washington, D.C.: Nervous and Mental Disease Pub. Co., 1927).

47. Walter Bromberg, "Mental States in Chronic Encephalitis," *Psychiatric Quarterly* 23, no. 1 (January 1930): 194.

48. Walter Bromberg, "Case Presentation, Meeting, N.Y. Academy, May 14, 1929," *Archives of Neurology and Psychiatry* 23 (January 1930): 194.

49. See Theodore R. Robie, "The Investigation of the Oedipus and Homosexual Complexes in Schizophrenia," *Archives of Neurology and Psychiatry* 23 (January 1930): 194.

49. See Theodore R. Robie, "The Investigation of the Oedipus and Homosexual Complexes in Schizophrenia," *Psychiatric Quarterly* 1 (1927): 231; Leland E. Hinsie, "Analytic Treatment of a Neurotic Reaction, A Study in Symbolism," *Psychiatric Quarterly* 1 (1927): 5; and C. S. Wolff, "Thought Content in Catatonic Dementia Praecox," *Psychiatric Quarterly* 6 (1932): 504.

50. William A. White, *Forty Years of Psychiatry* (Washington, D.C.: Nervous and Mental Disease Pub. Co., 1933), p. 57.

51. Frankwood Williams, "Is There a Mental Hygiene?" *Psychoanalytic Quarterly* 1 (1932): 119.

52. Manfred Bleuler, "Schizophrenia, Review of the Works of Professor Eugen Bleuler," *Archives of Neurology and Psychiatry* 26 (1931): 610.

53. Franz Alexander, "Schizophrenia Process: Critical Considerations of Psychoanalytic Treatment," *Archives of Neurology and Psychiatry* 26 (1931): 814.

54. Frieda Fromm-Reichmann, *Principles of Intensive Psychotherapy* (Chicago, Ill.: University of Chicago Press, 1950).

55. Karl M. Menninger, *A Psychiatrist's World: Selected Papers,* ed. Bernard Hill (New York: Viking Press, 1959), p. 838.

56. John C. Burnham, "From Avant-Garde to Specialism: Psychoanalysis in America," *History of the Behavioral Sciences* 15 (1979): 128.

57. Ibid., p. 131.
58. Paul Roazen, *Freud and His Followers* (New York: Alfred A. Knopf, 1975), p. 299.
59. Quoted in George C. Ham, "Psychoanalysis and Medical Education," *Current Psychiatric Therapies* vol. 1 (New York: Grune & Stratton, 1961), pp. 125-30.
60. S. Ferenczi and Otto Rank, *The Development of Psychoanalysis,* trans. C. Newton, Nervous and Mental Disease Monograph Series, no. 4 (Washington, D.C.: Nervous and Mental Disease Pub. Co., 1925).

4

BELLEVUE AND BEYOND

OLD BELLEVUE

From 1879 to the turn of the century, the insane pavilion of Bellevue Hospital was a depository for the indigent insane of New York City. Attended spottily by alienists and neurologists of the stature of Charles Dana for thirty years, it became a psychiatric hospital in 1910, when Menas S. Gregory ran the service single-handedly. Gregory, whose Armenian surname of Bulgukian was supplanted (according to legend) by that of his sponsor, Judge Gregory of Albany, gained his first experience in pavilion "F" of the Albany General Hospital, the first psychopathic ward in an American general hospital. Over the years, as the number of mental patients increased, the hospital widened its domain under Gregory's guidance. Several buildings in the Bellevue courtyard— one, a two-story barracklike structure for alcoholics and the other, the original site of the pest house, later the prison ward—were converted for psychiatric use. When I joined the staff as a junior psychiatrist in 1930, diagnoses of the stream of disturbed New Yorkers brought to Bellevue's doors included acute psychoses, panic reactions, suicide attempts, intoxications, depressions, and neuroses in all stages of decompensation.

The process of examination and disposition was relatively simple: Each morning Dr. Gregory and his assistants, Dr. Sam Feigen, one of New York University's own, and later Dr. Loughran, an import from the immigration service on Ellis Island, would sweep through the wards, making a quick survey of the patients examined the day before by the junior psychiatrists. The brief résumé of the case written on the green commitment petition received a glance; a few questions were directed to the bewildered patient, and a decision made whether or not to commit to a state hospital. Other patients, not committable and hence outside the legal process, were turned over to the ward physician for discharge. Drug addicts were un-heard-of, but alcoholics, detoxified but bleary-eyed, were herded into the street after the usual admonitions were given, only to return within a few days through the revolving door. Patients suffering from transitory states were passed into the arms of relatives, referred to their family physicians, or occasionally transferred to private sanatoria.

The more disturbed patients were commonly treated with hydrotherapy, the cold pack, or the omnipotent H & M (hyoscine and morphine). When their excited phase subsided, a commitment paper was drawn up and taken to a judge downtown who, after a proxy hearing, signed the paper. Relatives were informed that the patients were to be "sent to the country," a euphemism for Manhattan State Hospital or Central Islip State Hospital on Long Island. Only a few medications were available to the doctors. Barbiturates, paraldehyde, tincture of deodorized opium, and choral hydrate were the standbys; restraint by camisole, the hydrotherapy tub, and the cold pack were the mechanical aids.

As the service grew, the increased activity outdistanced the older buildings. A new, seven-story structure, exclusively for psychiatric patients, was completed in 1932 at Dr. Gregory's insistence, Mayor Jimmy Walker's support, and the concurrence of psychiatric leaders throughout the city. Well planned, the hospital soon filled with patients, staff, research projects, students, and social workers. Gone was the leisurely air of old Gotham suggested by the older buildings with their curlicue cornices, high ceilings, and room-high windows. The setting was worthy of an O. Henry story of the little people in the city of four million. And such a story was indeed enacted in the admitting office, a nondescript room, tucked under the staircase of the ancient administration building and furnished with long-worn, overstuffed chairs, and a battered desk.

On a steamy July night about midnight, a young man on his way to the East River, which was a hundred yards from the office, walked in asking for help before he sought final solace from the river. As junior staff member, I held the night duty. He wanted to know if I could help. I listened: An expatriated Viennese, driven from his native city by the impending Anschüluss and taken to Montreal by a young Canadian wife who immediately left him, he had found his way to New York. Friendless in a strange country and without resources, he talked of his desperation. As he spun out his story during the early hours of the morning, in stilted but adequate English, his depression lifted. A few suggestions and reassurance helped him to find a menial job in a restaurant. Over the months he reported his rise to manager, anglicized his name, and happily entered the stream of working New Yorkers.

Another humid July evening, a year later, found Karl (he kept his first name) arrested for indecent exposure in Brooklyn by a zealous police officer. The city had suffered a sex crime wave, and young males idly walking the streets were fair game. Karl, his coat over his arm, insisted that he merely scratched an old, sweaty abdominal scar! The officer claimed he masturbated in public. Arrested but released on his own recognizance, he appeared in my office in great distress. "You saved my life once, you must do it again," he pleaded. Perplexed, I asked for time to concoct a plan to aid this distressed man. Next morning before I could develop a workable plan, he rushed into the office jubilantly holding a copy of *The Daily News*. In bold face type, the headline read: "Inspector DiMartini [his arresting officer and only witness] Dead of Heart Attack!"

The "New Hospital" Vitalized

To return to the new psychiatric hospital, its increased activity was further enlivened by the importation in 1930 of Paul Schilder from the University of Vienna via the Phipps Institute, as clinical director and research professor of psychiatry at New York University. Under Schilder's stimulus, ward rounds attained the status of university conferences and research projects eventuated in important papers. For more than a decade, until Schilder's untimely death, the period of creative research in many fields escalated.

With the expansion of services, my assignment moved from the acute wards with their unmanageable manics and withdrawn schizophrenics, the everlasting M & H and cold packs, to the children's ward. New vistas in human behavior opened. Children's problems extended from hysterical reactions to autism, from organic defects to acting-out behavior. Treatment of such a heterogenous group proved difficult. On a hunch I organized a courtroom scene with the children as jury, myself as judge, and the nurses as prosecuting and defending attorneys—a kind of psychodrama. Misbehavior became the issue to be judged by the peers of patient-miscreants. Soon the juvenile jury not only gave pronouncements of social guilt but offered dynamic explanations of misbehavior, for example, "He hates the hospital"; "She don't like her foster mother." It was revealing to observe how easily children accepted the meaning of maladjustment to socio-pyschological realities.

This type of rudimentary play therapy was valuable in differentiating autistic or organic problems from neurotic disturbances among children. Later Lauretta Bender, who succeeded me on the children's service, extended these group activities and techniques to puppet shows.[1] The problem of autistic children, which was initially studied by Leo Kanner at Johns Hopkins, led Bender to analyze spontaneous motility and its disorders among children. Her method, which led to the Bender-Gestalt test, at its outset involved placing chalk on the sidewalks of the city streets, allowing children to spontaneously draw what they wished, and then studying how scrawls eventuated in characteristic designs.[2] Motility patterns thus induced in normal children then were brought into relation with those of catatonic schizophrenics and other organic conditions.[3] Other studies, such as the development of the Goodenough test by Karen Machover, a clinical psychologist, evolved from their original aim to measure intellectual levels to illumination of the body image thus became invaluable evaluative instruments. The draw-a-person test, which started with the children, in Machover's hands grew to be a ready source of personality analysis of all types of patients.[4]

This group of studies, covering the child's perceptual progress in building a social and real world, formed part of Schilder's constructive psychiatry.[5] He had suggested that not only motility but also such abstractions as "time" were modalities used by children in developing their enlarged world image. This genetic view of a child's social ego growth, a fascinating concept, became the basis for a research project to test the meaning of time among children.[6] Using normal and neurotic subjects, I questioned children in simple terms—"How old is an old man?" "What does time mean?" Included in the group were both gifted and defective children. The answers were concrete and derived from objective rather than subjective experiences. "Time is numbers on a clock," said a five-year-old child. "Time is to get out of bed," said another. "An old man is skinny; he don't eat much, can't move fast . . . , and dies," reported a seven-year-old retarded child.

It was extraordinary how under Schilder's encouragement almost every clinical problem encountered on the wards became grist for the research mill. Many of the staff carried their research *Trieb* through their professional lives. Bender elaborated on childhood schizophrenia[7]; David Wechsler, the chief psychologist, laboriously developed his Bellevue-Wechsler adult intelligence test under the Works Progress Administration funding of the Roosevelt administration; Sam Parker, a former student of Stekel in Vienna, continued to work with Schilder[8]; and Frank Curran enlarged the field of adolescent behavior problems.[9] The stimulus for innovation flowed in diverse clinical directions; from Frederic Wertham of "catathymic crisis" fame; Nathaniel Ross, training psychoanalyst; Ralph Brancale, criminologist; David Impastato, pioneer in electroshock therapy; Sylvan Keiser, teaching analyst; Irving Bieber, the leader of a group initiating the analytic treatment of homosexuals; John Frosch, editor of the annual *Psychoanalytic Yearbook*; Helen Yarnell, the author of an original book on firesetters; Milton Abeles with studies in amnesia; Morris Herman, originally an internist; and Joseph Wortis, who introduced insulin shock treatment. The staff's productions, however, were miniscule compared to Schilder's output. Lectures, books, papers, and discussions at scientific meetings rolled out in prodigious quantity. His drive had been lifelong. Fritz Wittels once reminded us that Freud had faintly remonstrated with Schilder in Vienna because his work covered "too wide dimensions."

The Schilderian Influence

Besides his broad background in physiological neuropsychiatry, Schilder introduced the staff to philosophy in the form of phenomenology. This development of Edmund Husserl's had already taken a strong hold on philosophy in Europe. Its application to clinical problems was unique, for it served as a keystone for Schilder's *Constructive Psychiatry.*

In brief, phenomenology supplanted metaphysics, the reigning posture of late nineteenth-century philosophers. It clashed with idealism in its insistence that the "mind" should be analyzed through the immediacy of experiencing without reasoning, deduction, or induction. In effect this meant dealing with perception as primary clinical-experimental material. In the words of Marvin Farber,[10] a close student of Husserl, phenomenology strove to supplant previous philosophic thinking by forming an "autonomous discipline . . . a rigorous science of philosophy," the basic premise of which was analysis of experience per se.[11]

Because it was extremely foreshortened, the philosophic background for Schilder's experimentation was not easy for those trained in a clinical tradition to grasp. We gradually absorbed the meaning of his philosophic *Anlage* through the research projects to which many of the staff turned. The man and his ideas functioned as an automatic stimulus. As a man and as a clinical leader, Schilder was impossible to dislike. A slightly built man, his coal-black eyes and hair reminded one of a Turk rather than the Europeanized Viennese we had encountered among other expatriates. He exuded a true *Gemütlickeit* without stodginess; wit and urbanity without affectation. His *joie de vivre* covered a mind whose penetration and uniqueness reminded one of Einstein's.

The usual way of regarding clinical things could be turned on end in a moment to achieve a totally different, and equally valid, Gestalt. This gift of perceiving hitherto unseen Gestalts was said to have lain behind the discovery of the Schilder-Foix disease, *Encephalitis Periaxialis Diffusa.* Legend has it that Schilder diagnosed the condition in one case with one microscopic slide of that case, and I venture to add, probably one glance at that slide. Similarly, his feelings could be expressed in one-liners: When Adolf Meyer questioned his tremendous scientific output, Schilder remarked smilingly, "If you don't publish, you're autistic." In his teachings he displayed an unusual acquaintance with psychological, psycho-physiological, and psychoanalytical literature, but he was unafraid to depart from Freudianism when logic and methodology were in question. Fritz Wittels called him a "Faustian man who worked without rest and without strain in many fields."[12] Yet Schilder's wide interests and flashes of intuition in relating disparate facts of an organic and psychic nature did not escape criticism. For example, in his 1938 book *Psychotherapy,* which was reviewed by Abraham Myerson, he was taken to task for stating, "When a person suffers by organic disease, there is no need for further punishment, and he may be relieved from his feeling of guilt."[13] This, like other statements, Myerson complained, "assert much and prove little or nothing."[14] In general, Myerson thought Schilder lacked "that essential humility before the unknown and unprovable, which should govern scientific . . . statements." Criticism of this type, however, did not deter Schilder.

As the staff became involved in research under Schilder's direction, the problem of how to relate living experiences (phenomenology) with the Freudian unconscious arose. Schilder's plan involved studying subjective perceptions among healthy persons as well as cortically injured persons displaying agnosias and aphasias. By studying perception among healthy and cortically handicapped persons, he could follow the development of the body images that underlay preconscious and unconscious constructions. In conjunction with Leo Kanner in Baltimore, he started with experiments on visual perception to establish how the body image, the postural model (Henry Head) of the body, evolved out of the perceptions of each of the five senses. Experiments of visual perception were followed with those of hearing with Sam Parker at Bellevue and then touch and smell with myself; the fifth sense, taste, was not completed.

Schilder's technique in this group of experiments can be illustrated by those techniques of the tactile perception experiments on which I worked. The experiments were aimed eventually at understanding the symptomatology of psychotic and neurotic conditions, as they combined psychic (unconscious) motivation and the individual perceptual background. The tactile experiments started with volunteers from the staff and student group who were asked to report their preception of long-lasting touches on the hand.[15] These reports were charted, and the same experiments were then attempted with the subject in a Barany rotating chair in order to observe the effect of vestibular irritation on perception. Our results demonstrated that when sensations are attended to, that is, their subjective effect observed by the subject, they represented more than a static, one-time experience. Perception of sensations moved, fragmented, diffused on the skin. A body image built of various perceptions, then, was not a unitary image but a shifting, moving one, ordinarily suppressed by healthy persons. The perceptions indeed had a life of their own. In illnesses, toxic states (alcoholism, drug intoxication), or functional psychoses (schizophrenia), these disintegration products were elaborated into illusions, hallucinations, and paraesthesias, which were interwoven with unconscious ideation, sexual fantasies, fears, or panic reactions. The conclusion was inescapable: Distortions of body image lay at the base of many psychotic conditions, as well as neurotic symptomatology, an example of the juncture of psycho-physiological factors.[16] In the case of toxic psychoses, such as delirium tremens, the characteristic "little people, pink elephants, and mocking green dwarfs," represented merely dramatizations of visual and tactile products of perceptual decay. The same technique employed in studying olfactory sensation produced similar results.[17] In effect, the influence of distorted body image due to toxic substances (alcohol, for example) in union with unconscious anxieties explained many bizarre symptoms on a physiological-psychological basis. This type of holistic interpretation seemed more complete than any purely psychological theory that had been advanced up to that time.

New vistas opened up by Schilder's concept of "ideologies," some of which were abstract like time, some of which were personal like death and sex, which tied individual attitudes to the common feelings society offers. Using the questionnaire method, he explored subjective feelings in these areas, starting from an intuitive position that opposed Freud's notion of an unconscious death instinct, thanatos, the polar opposite of libido. This metaphysical abstractions—that the end result of human instinctual life was a winding-down to rest, or entropy—seemed contradictory to actual experience. Schilder saw the goal of human striving to be continued ego satisfaction. "How," he asked, "aside from theoretical constructs, did people actually perceive their own, or other's death?'' To answer the question, we developed an elaborate questionnaire that concerned the individual's fantasies, experiences, fears, and hopes about death and dying.

The questionnaires were offered to psychology students from Columbia and New York universities and to patients in the hospital. The conclusions we reached from the questionnaires indicated that attitudes toward death inevitably represented something wanted from life. The attitudes toward death evoked from normal and mentally ill persons indicated that the fantasy of dying meant real things in life—an escape from unbearable situations, a means of forcing affection from others, the satisfaction of masochistic fantasies, a picture of one's final narcissistic perfection in death and so on. Schilder and I concluded the long paper, which was published in the *Psychoanalytic Review* in 1933, with the statement: "All libidinous roads lead to death, and death becomes thus the perfect symbol of life."[18] The paper was presented at a meeting of the American Psychiatric Association in Atlantic City that year, but it made little impression on our colleagues. Now, forty years later, psychotherapists deal freely with the images and fantasies of death among incurable patients, trying to soften their anguish.

That Schilder denied the death wish theory was characteristic of him, for experience and living—existentialism and phenomenology—comprised the essence of his philosophy. Psychiatry became to Schilder a biopsychosocial undertaking. His papers and books were not always easy to understand; sometimes repetitious, even obscure, they nevertheless were aimed at a holistic therapy that was not always appreciated by the psychiatric community of the 1930s. Still, he used analytic concepts freely, approving of Freudianism but not idolatrous of it. Perhaps it was this attitude of his that lay behind the New York Psychoanalytic Society's rejection of him for membership when he was voted down nineteen to eighteen. The vote was greeted with consternation in some quarters: Jelliffe, for one, exploded in anger. He exclaimed, "A fresh voice in psychiatry excluded by the orthodox!" It was no secret that Schilder, while a member of the Vienna Psychoanalytic Society, had "found the society stifling and did not passively surrender to Freud."[19] Recognizing this trait in Schilder, which I suspect Jelliffe secretly admired, he vented his spleen by commenting on the anal obstinancy of those who had opposed Schilder's admission to the society. Rumor had it that Lawrence Kubie, a neurophysiologist at Columbia and later at Yale, then currently a member of the New York Psychoanalytic Society, had cast the deciding negative vote. In any event, Schilder did not follow the orthodox line of five sessions a week, a passive stance maintained by the analyst, no physical interactions with patients (physical examinations or prescribing medication), use of a couch, reliance on interpretations, and no direct advice to the patient.

THE REVISIONISTS

In spite of this accepted formula for analysis, signs of differing emphasis were becoming visible. We heard of the Washington-Baltimore group, of Clara Thompson and Harry Stack Sullivan's interpersonal relationship therapy in which the analyst did not remain an impersonal voice somewhere behind the patient but rather came into closer relation as a "participant observer" of the patient's reactions. This more realistic and medical posture of the therapist made sense, even though Sullivan's language and innovations (for example, "parataxic phenomenon" in place of "transference") tended to be obscure and convoluted. Sullivan's methods breathed a spirit of American pragmatism into psychotherapy in contrast to the metapsychological subtleties of orthodox analysis.

Beyond these deviations, the conflict among the pioneers, Freud, Adler, and Jung, added piquancy to those who witnessed the analytic scene from a ringside seat. Other than reading bits of Jung's works, which were considered too esoteric for clinical minds, our generation had no opportunity to see or hear this sage. There were fewer Jungian analysts in New York than Adlerian therapists. One evening, however, an opportunity arose to hear of the growing schism among analysts at a private meeting arranged at the Academy of Medicine. Dr. Esther Harding, a Jungian, was invited to present her method of analysis to a small group that included Brill, Jelliffe, Oberndorf, and a few neophytes. The meeting was an informal session in a smaller room and intended as an intimate exchange of scientific confidences. After a polite social skirmish, Dr. Harding, a scholarly looking woman with a pince-nez, began her account of her patient's analysis according to Jungian principles. She began with an involved dream the patient had brought to her: He had been on a mountain top; there was an explosion and a large figure emerged. Harding analyzed this figure as an archetype belonging to the collective unconscious. Everyone listened intently, but I noticed Brill becoming tense and restless, while Jelliffe drummed his fingers on the table. A sense of impatience pervaded the room. Finally, Brill, unable to contain himself any longer, burst out: "I can make nothing of these symbols. . . . This has nothing to do with analysis." Oberndorf said a few things calculated to calm the waters, but it was clear the schism could never be breached.

Contact with Alfred Adler was less frigid. The staff had a chance at a Mount Sinai Hospital conference to hear Adler in person. In a routinized manner, he lectured on his individual psychology. A stocky man, comfortably dressed, and exuding the *Gemütlich* of his native Vienna, he spoke in a gentle manner of the development of inferiority feelings in the child, the total "life plan" of the individual, and the very human "will to dominate." Avoiding the intricate metapsychology of orthodox psychoanalysis, Adler dwelled on the simple drives and frustrations that gave rise to neurosis. His relatively uncomplicated system of viewing the origin of human conflicts made sense, but it lacked the dramatic flair, the mythological symbolism and prurient fascination with the submerged sexual life of Freudianism. His gentle, almost offhand manner, like a tired teacher speaking to a group of students, gave no hint of the bitterness that had attended Freud's reaction to Adlerian psychology or his response thereto. "Individual Psychology," wrote Freud, "had very little to do with psychoanalysis. . . . [It] leads to a parasitic existence. . . . Its very name is inappropriate and seems to have been the product of embarrassment."[20] Adler replied, "Psychoanalysis is filth."[21] Freud retorted, "I made a pygmy great."[22]

There were technical bases for this vicious conflict: Adler claimed the discovery of urethral erotism and the character trait of ambition. Freud insisted it was his own idea. Adler dwelt on the "will to power" behind the neurosis; Freud wrote, "His [Adler's] writings are belles lettres rather than scientific writings." The struggle, some two decades old, was less vigorously echoed in America, but the psychoanalytic group in New York, at least, regarded Adlerian psychology as superficial and "oversimplified."[23]

Those outside psychoanalytic circles who heard of Jung-Freud conflicts were not as derisive of Jung as were the hard-liners. The Jung deviation occasioned little animosity among those who sat in the penumbra of analysis, although it was agreed that Jung's work lay on a level other than psychoanalysis. The concept of collective unconscious and his interest in mythology, alchemy, and the primitive archetypes—*animus* and *anima*—seemed too poetical and mystical for therapeutically oriented analysts. Acknowledging that Jung's word association test was a valuable psychological implement, whatever else we read of Jung fell into the category of psychiatric history, an interesting but impractical serendipity.[24] The English analyst Edward Glover expressed the common attitude toward Jung's analytical psychology when he wrote, "The key to the riddle of Jung's psychology is that Jung is a conscious psychologist. . . . His psychology has no relation to Freudian psychology. The most implicit, but often explicit, tendency of his theories is to prove Freud's discovery of the unconscious . . . inaccurate, totally false or totally unnecessary. . . . This is Jung's consuming passion."[25] There wasn't more to say. Beyond that dictum, Jung's alleged support of the Nazi movement in Germany did little to endear him to American psychiatrists. All these events occurred in the first triad of the 1930s. But other more pressing problems engaged our attention.

Beginnings in Social Psychiatry

Psychiatric activity in hospitals and in literature did not abate the gloom that covered the city and nation during these years. Industry and business were stifled by the Great Depression. Money was scarce, jobs impossible to get, luxuries forgotten. The confidence of the roaring twenties faded to an omnipresent sense of defeatism. Doctors' incomes from practice became practically non-existent. Long bread lines included men of substance, shocked by the experience of being unwanted by business and industry. Men sold apples on street corners at five cents each and waited for President Hoover's promise that the country would soon "turn the corner." Professionals like the engineers who designed the New York subways were glad to get work as manual laborers; lawyers sold neckties door-to-door. The Works Progress Administration developed "make work" for factory hands, writers, dramatists, and mechanics, while the specter of the dole shook New York and the rest of the country to its roots. The bank holiday closure of 1932 increased the general insecurity in spite of President Roosevelt's ringing anodyne, "There is nothing to fear but fear itself." A diffuse anxiety that amounted to widespread demoralization (the "dole neurosis" the English called it) made individual psychoanalytical treatment appear to be an out-of-reach luxury.

Out of this matrix of anxiety that called for therapy, group therapy appeared as a practical solution. There had been a few pioneers in America who had experimented with a type of group therapy for some years. Edward Lazell at Saint Elizabeth's Hospital in Washington, D.C. had lectured in 1919 to mental patients, explaining the meaning of depression, hallucinations, and inferiority feelings.[26] Trigant Burrow, a little later, worked with groups in which the self-image of one person interacted with the self-image of another within the group.[27] Louis Wender at the Hastings Hillside Hospital in Tarrytown, New York, an outgrowth of the Jewish Mental Health Society of which Israel Strauss was president and prime mover, introduced group therapy between 1928 and 1930, instructing his patients in an informal way of familiar emotional patterns, sibling rivalry, identification, transference reactions, castration anxiety, and such like.[28]

Simultaneously at Bellevue, Schilder formed groups of six or seven patients from the outpatient clinic. He approached them tentatively, first requesting an autobiography written by the patient "with nothing held back."[29] The life history was then brought before the group with the therapist acting as a leader; interpretations were made and similarities to other patients' histories discussed. This technique represented a transition from psychoanalytical treatment since the group members also were seen individually twice a week. As a commentary on the social climate of the times (1936 to 1940), Schilder avoided "mixing the sexes in the group . . . except for the occasional female patient . . . analyzed for a long time." This modest disclaimer notwithstanding, the staff and some patients were temporarily shocked to hear a patient's open descriptions of his sexual practices. From this unusual technique, Schilder went on to present questionnaires covering such subjects as the individual's attitudes toward other persons, his or her own body, social contacts, and such like. These attitudes, imbedded in the individual's personality, he called "ideologies." The method of questionnaires, which usually was employed by psychologists and sociologists, was frowned on by the medical fraternity. Nevertheless, Schilder persevered. His aim was to bring social attitudes into relation with neuroses, a reflection of Karen Horney's view that social influences were basic in the formation of personality.

In the hands of a few pioneers, group therapy in the 1930s carried a faddish and unscientific connotation among therapists, particularly those of the analytic persuasion. The discussion of life problems among patients in a group and the later inclusion of the leader as both a participant and an observer stimulated a queasy feeling among psychiatrists. When Jacob Moreno brought his psychodrama to New York, criticism first greeted his methods, then grudging acceptance. As much sociological as psychiatric, Moreno's approach had been stimulated years earlier by the liberal-socialistic atmosphere of Vienna and the experimental theatre movement of Stanislavsky. This atmosphere that pervaded the 1920s was characterized by historians as "one of the most fertile, original and creative periods in art, architecture, music, literature, and psychology" in postwar Vienna.[30] Initially beginning as an impromptu theater, where actors spontaneously played out themes from their own private worlds, the theater of spontaneity eventually became therapeutic.[31] By manipulating the actor and the audience into reversing roles, developing "mirror images" of each other, Moreno claimed the essential encounters between two or more human beings could be brought to the surface. Moreno's technique involved the direct opposite of the privacy of the usual therapeutic dyad. As he prodded his player-patients to see themselves in each other's eyes, public exposure of individual emotional problems seemed to reduce embarrassment; a sense of human unity arose. Family situations enacted on the stage were real: Anger, irritation, the shock of recognition of oneself in the "mirror" reversal produced a profound effect. The several sessions I witnessed with their immediate catharsis seemed genuine. But it wasn't until years later that I became a group therapist; for the moment an activist approach to therapy appeared both plausible and effective.

Moreno called his psychodrama the third psychiatric revolution, since it rested not upon the minority of mental patients but upon the "normal group," that is, society itself, with its personal interrelations and emotional cross fire.[32] In particular, Moreno's methods bypassed the unconscious as a prime object of attention and passed to interactionism, the "here and now" of the patient's emotional front. The criticisms of psychodrama, which was sometimes performed before audiences of several hundred, centered on Moreno's strident claim of the "passing of the psychoanalytic system."[33] His attack on the Freudian system did not go unanswered: Some bewailed the "pitfall that lurks in the coequal relationship between therapist and patient. . . . The therapist has been trained to understand . . . emotional disorders, whereas, the patient has not."[34] At the time, group therapy and psychodrama, considered an eccentric import from Europe, remained interesting but unproven methods of psychotherapy.

And Beyond

Not adverse to straying from orthodoxy, I wandered into other nonsanctioned arenas such as the phyloanalysis of Trigant Burrow. Charles Thompson, a colleague at Bellevue, a dignified Baltimorean, had suggested that phyloanalysis might open up new vistas. Accordingly, I visited the Lifwyn Foundation, located in a brownstone house near lower Park Avenue in New York, where Burrow and his associates lived and worked. The atmosphere was lowkeyed, the persuasion gentle, and the discussion without hint of rancor. Originally a member of one of the elite group that had organized the American Psychoanalytic Association in 1911, Burrow had developed a theory that the social tensions between individuals that might eventuate in neurosis were phyletic in that such tensions involved the human race, hence phyloanalysis. He claimed with development of languages, semantic symbols took the place of instincts in communication; conflicts, therefore, centered around language communications instanced by tensions located in the forehead. Such conflicts were the "symbolic" representations of antagonism between humans.[35] Burrow's therapy was based on his rather abstruse theory of obtaining "consensual validation" between neurotic patients and therapists to neutralize those social "tensions." He had arrived at this formulation when a patient on the couch in a classical analysis said, "If you were in my position would you feel as I do? Why don't we change places?" Burrow agreed and thus obtained a different view of the therapeutic transaction.

Burrow's theory of neurosis and consequent therapy occasioned little interest chiefly because of its abstruse premise: "[Neurosis] is an error of our mental refraction. . . . We assume pictorial rather than real relationship to others."[36] Burrows explained, "Man has an unreal apperception of his fellows . . . and consequent false inferences," the cure of which was a "consensual validation" of this relation. I confess phyloanalysis was beyond my comprehension. In a review in the *Journal of Orthopsychiatry,* I called his school of psychotherapy "too close to transcendentalism" to be of clinical value. In retrospect, however, Burrow's criticism of the "dogmatic, complacent, authoritarian tendencies of psychiatrists" was not without value, although his conclusion that neurosis lay upon a phylogenetic base appealed to few. In a review of Burrow's works, Professor Thomas Eliot of Notherwestern University rejected his views as "mystical and religious in a Buddhistic sense."[37]

It became apparent to me that variations in psychotherapy had both a long history and a vigorous present life. Pastoral psychiatry, which was then in a period of rebirth, was being dispensed by Spencer Cowles, the son of a distinguished Boston psychiatrist of the turn of the century. Dr. Cowles's out-patient clinic was the venerable Saint Mark's-in-the-Bowery Church, a structure that dated back to the New York of Revolutionary days. The body-and-Soul Clinic, headed by Spencer Cowles, ran on semireligious lines. It was a vivid example of pastoral psychiatry, which was then attaining a respectable stance in psychotherapy. There had been attempts, many successful, during the first three decades of the century, to utilize religious faith in treating and managing neuroses. The Emmanuel movement of the turn of the century tried to combine psychology with religious ministering. Cowles's clinic added a new factor, the presence of Smiley Blanton, a well-trained psychoanalyst and psychiatrist. He worked with the patients psychologically, while Cowles and later Norman Vincent Peale of the Marble Collegiate Church on Fifth Avenue in New York, dispensed religious solace.[38] In contrast to this staid atmosphere, Saint Mark's-in-the-Bowery partook of the turmoil and poverty of the East Side. The meetings were open to the public, and Dr. Cowles, standing at a lecturn with two converging purple shafts of light illuminating his figure, would speak to the audience, explaining in simple terms how psychological conflicts eventuated in neuroses.

Contact with the byways of psychotherapy gave one a perspective: Prior to and concomitant with scientific psychotherapy practiced by medically educated men and women were methods of healing from most disparate sources. Was there a common element in these diverse techniques and theories? William A. White had mentioned the common thread of "hope" in a symposium on therapy in schizophrenia in 1931.[39] Was hope and belief an epiphenomenon or the basic mechanisms in the therapeutic transaction? With this thought in mind, I gathered all types of psychotherapy into a history entitled *The Mind of Man, The Story of Man's Conquest of Mental Illness* under the assumption that prescientific and scientific methods enjoyed some—though unequal—successes.[40]

THE FIELD ENLARGES

By the middle of the 1930s, that burgeoning plant, psychiatry, had grown into a sturdy tree with a massive trunk and solid branches, some adorned with palatable and nourishing fruits, some unproductive or overgrown with flamboyant offshoots. The center of psychiatric research no longer clung to the East Coast. Although the giants of neuropsychiatry worked in Boston, New York,

Philadelphia, Baltimore, and Washington, D.C.; centers in the Midwest, the Plain States, and the West Coast, were producing ideas and investigating clinical problems, as well as writing, teaching, and publishing.

No branch of psychiatry was left untouched or uninvestigated. Organic problems from Alzheimer's disease to gliosis in the choreic brain, from treatment of schizophrenia with carbon dioxide, Amytal, cyanide compounds, and oxygen to discussions of constitutional factors in homosexuality filled the pages of the *American Journal of Psychiatry*.[41] The variety of subjects in the journals and addresses before the scientific audiences was astounding. Some were in the direction of psychiatric growth, some proved to be trivial. A scrutiny of the journal's pages during the early 1930s indicates a rising interest in psychosomatic medicine (H. Flanders Dunbar on emotions and bodily change) and in clinical studies (Elizabeth Bryan on neologisms), experimental reports on chemical changes (John Whitehorn on blood sugar changes in emotional states), biochemical treatment methods in depression, and so forth.[42] Published studies were becoming more exacting; therapeutic ideas more closely watched, as in Arthur P. Noyes's article in which he refuted the applicability of psychoanalytic treatment in state hospitals in favor of "listening to patients, re-education and suggestion."[43] The meetings of the American Psychiatric Association were well attended. The energetic Dr. Clarence Charles Burlingame, who was chairman for public education in the association, reported a "definite quickening of interest in psychiatry throughout the nation."[44]

This quickening interest was not confined to professional circles. Literature, the theatre, and the cinema reflected the more stable position of psychiatry, especially psychoanalysis, among the public. Earlier scoffings at Freudianism, for example in Susan Glaspell's 1917 play *Suppressed Desires* in which the hero, Stephen Brewster, is analyzed to B-rewster (rooster), were replaced by Eugene O'Neill's productions at the Provincetown Playhouse.[45] His play *Great God Brown* in 1926, which employed symbolism and free association, as did *Strange Interlude* in 1928, led critic Alexander Woolcott to dub him the "unbridled Eugene O'Neill."[46] In 1941 *Lady in the Dark* by Moss Hart featured Gertrude Lawrence, who played the part of a troubled lady undergoing psychoanalysis.[47] The play was a theatrical success and attuned to a New York audience. Brooks Atkinson, drama critic of the *New York Times*, commented in tones of muted admiration, "[Its theme] was one to explore and express."[48] Few literary critics disputed the fact that the changed direction and content of literature in America followed "depth psychology . . . [and] the prevailing scientific climate of ideas." The open sesame of the "inherent drama of the subconscious" led to a populous world of psychologic novels from 1920 onward.[49]

NOTES

1. See Lauretta Bender, "Group Activities on a Children's Ward as a Method of Psychotherapy." *American Journal of Psychiatry* 43, no. 5 (March 1937): 192; and L. Bender and A. G. Woltmann, ::Use of Puppet Shows as a Psychotherapeutic Method for Behavior Problems in Children," *American Journal of Orthopsychiatry* 6 (1936): 341.

2. L. Bender, "Gestalt Principles of Sidewalk Drawings and Games of Children," *Journal of Genetic Psychology* 41 (1932): 192-210.

3. Walter Bromberg, "Schizophrenic-like Psychoses in Defective Children," *American Journal of Psychiatry* 90 (1934): 226.

4. Karen Machover, *Personality Projection in the Drawing of a Human Figure* (Springfield, Ill.: Charles Thomas, 1949).

5, Paul Schilder, *Contributions to Developmental Psychology,* ed. Lauretta Bender (New York: International University Press, 1936), chap. 3, p. 61 et seq.

6. Walter Bromberg, "The Meaning of Time for Children," *American Journal of Orthopsychiatry* 8 (1938): 142.

7. Lauretta Bender, "Childhood Schizophrenia," *American Journal of Orthopsychiatry* 17 (1947): 40.

8. Sam Parker and P. Schilder, "Acoustic Imagination and Acoustic Hallucinations," *Archives of Neurology and Psychiatry* 34 (1935): 744.

9. Frank J. Curran and P. Schilder, "A Constructive Approach to the Problems of Childhood and Adolescence," *Journal of Criminal Psychopathology* 2 (1940): 125.

10. Marvin Farber, *The Foundation of Phenomenology* (Albany, N.Y.: State University of New York Press, 1967), p. 19.

11. Walter Bromberg, *Paul Schilder, Mind Explorer,* ed. Donald Shaskas and William Roller (to be published in 1983).

12. Fritz Wittels, "In Memoriam, Paul Schilder," *Psychoanalytic Quarterly* 10 (1941): 131.

13. Paul Schilder, *Psychotherapy* (New York: W. W. Norton & Co., 1938), p. 32.

14. A. Myerson, book review, *American Journal of Psychiatry* 95 (March 1939): 1251.

15. Walter Bromberg and Paul Schilder, "On Tactile Imagination and Tactile After-Effects," *Journal of Nervous and Mental Disease* 76 no. 1 (July 1932): 37.

16. Walter Bromberg and Paul Schilder, "Psychologic Considerations in Alcoholic Hallucinosis: Castration and Dismemberment Motives," *International Journal of Psychoanalysis* 14 (1933): 206.

17. Walter Bromberg and Paul Schilder, "Olfactory Imagination and Olfactory Hallucinations," *Archives of Neurology and Psychiatry* 32 (September 1934): 467.

18. Walter Bromberg and Paul Schilder, "Death and Dying," *Psychoanalytic Review* 20 (1933): 133.

19. Paul Roazen, *Freud and his Followers* (New York: Alfred A. Knopf, 1975), p. 335.

20. Sigmund Freud, *New Introductory Lectures on Psychoanalysis*, trans. W. J. Sprott (New York: W. W. Norton, Co., 1933), p. 140.

21. Roazen, *Freud and his Followers,* p. 210.

22. Ibid.

23. A. Kardiner, Personal communication, 1937.

24. C. G. Jung, *Contributions to Analytical Psychology*, trans. H. G. Baynes and C. F. Baynes (New York: The Bollingen Foundation, 1928).

25. Edward Glover, *Freud or Jung* (New York: W. W. Norton; London: Allen & Unwin, 1950).

26. E. W. Lazell, "The Group Treatment of Dementia Praecox," *Psychoanalytic Review* 8 (1921): 168.

27. Trigant Burrow, "The Group Method of Analysis," *Psychoanalytic Review* 14 (1927): 268.

28. Louis Wender, "Group Psychotherapy: A Study of Its Application," *Psychiatric Quarterly* 14 (1940): 708.

29. Paul Schilder, *Psychotherapy,* rev. ed. by L. Bender (New York: W. W. Norton, 1950), p. 203 et seq.

30. Allan Toulmin and Stephen Toulmin, *Wittgenstein's Vienna* (New York: Simon & Schuster, 1973), p. 9.

31. Jacob L. Moreno, *The Theatre of Spontaneity,* trans. J. Moreno (New York: Beacon House, 1923).

32. Jacob Moreno and Zerka Moreno, *Psychodrama, Foundations of Psychotherapy,* 2 vols. (New York: Beacon House, 1959), 2:104.

33. Jules Masserman, "Functions of the Unconscious," in *Psychodrama, Foundations of Psychotherapy,* p. 60.

34. J. B. Wheelwright, "Functions of the Unconscious," in *Psychodrama, Foundations of Psychotherapy,* p. 78.

35. Trigant Burrow, "Psychoanalysis in Theory and in Life," *Journal of Nervous and Mental Disease* 64, no. 3 (September 1926): 209.

36. Trigant Burrow, "A Relative Concept of Consciousness: An Analysis of Consciousness in its Ethnic Origin," *Psychoanalytic Review* 12, no. 1 (1925): 1.

37. Thomas D. Eliot, "Review of the Social Philosophy of Trigant Burrow," *Mental Hygiene* 12 no. 3 (July 1928): 530.

38. Smiley Blanton and Norman V. Peale, *Faith is the Answer* (New York: Prentice-Hall, 1941).

39. William A. White, "Discussion," *American Journal of Psychiatry* 88 (1931): 514.

40. Walter Bromberg, *The Mind of Man: The Story of Man's Conquest of Mental Illness* (New York: Harper & Bros., 1937).

41. See F. H. Gildea et al., "Comparative Study of Changes Produced by Various Drugs in Schizophrenic Patients," *American Journal of Psychiatry* 91 (May 1935): 1289; and George W. Henry and Hugh M. Galbraith, "Constitutional Factors in Homosexuality," *American Journal of Psychiatry* 91 (May 1934): 1247.

42. Flanders H. Dunbar, "Problems of Convalescence and Chronic Illness, A Preliminary Discussion," *American Journal of Psychiatry* 92 (March 1936): 1095; Elizabeth L. Bryan. "Forty Cases Exhibiting Neologisms," *American Journal of Psychiatry* 90 (November 1933): 579; and John C. Whitehorn, "Blood Sugar in Relation to Emotional Reactions," *American Journal of Psychiatry* 91 (May 1934): 987.

43. Arthur P. Noyes, "Psychotherapy in State Hospitals," *American Journal of Psychiatry* 91 (May 1935): 1353.

44. "News and Comments," *American Journal of Psychiatry* 92 (May 1936): 1461.

45. Susan Glaspell and George Cram Cook, *Suppressed Desires* (Provincetown Players, 1917).

46. *On Stage,* ed. Bernard Beckman and Howard Seigman (New York: Arno Press, New York Times Co., Quadrangle, 1956), p. 63.

47. Ibid., p. 14.

48. Cleanth Brooks, et al., eds., *American Literature: The Makers and Making* (New York: St. Martin's Press, 1973), p. 1149.

49. *Encyclopedia Americana,* International ed., s.v. "American Literature," Section IV, "The 20th Century Authors."

5
PSYCHIATRY ENTERS CRIMINOLOGY

Crime and delinquency had already attracted mental hygienists, who felt that they were appropriate fields for preventive efforts. The rapid strides that were being made in understanding personality formation led to the hope that the findings of psychopathology might illuminate the criminal mind and show the way to the treatment of criminals. Psychiatric progress rode on the wings of the reform movement, which sought to bring criminals out of the class of benighted men doomed to eternal pariahship into a class of individual offenders who were worthy of psychological study. Already the issue of mental deficiency had been tested. Whereas Charles Goring, working with the prison population in England in 1913 found "the one vital mental constitutional factor in the etiology of crime is defective intelligence," examination of American convicts in the following decade yielded a different result.[1] In 1928, after psychological testing, Carl Murchison found his criminal group to be superior in intelligence to the white draft group of World War I that he had also tested.[2] As studies in this area progressed, it became clear that feeblemindedness was less significant as the vital element in criminal behavior than "neuropathic or psychopathic" defects. Attention then turned to the criminal as a human being with a body, a mind, and a personal history.

During the Roaring Twenties with its racketeers and professional extoritionists spawned by the Prohibition era, the public was little interested in psychiatry's effort to understand the offender's personality and ego structure. They had experienced the "battle of experts" in insanity cases before the courts, and they were alternately amused and incensed by the insanity defense. Since the days of McNaghten the press and its readers had seen the battling alienists in an unsavory light. No less a personage than Queen Victoria had blasted the counselors and alienists when McNaghten was acquitted by reason of insanity of killing the prime minister's secretary in 1843. Her majesty inveighed against the lawyers "[who] advise the Jury to pronounce the verdict of Not Guilty on account of Insanity, when everybody is morally convinced that . . . [he] is perfectly conscious and aware of what he did."[3]

Queen Victoria's complaint was echoed by jurists and laymen in America for the remainder of the century. They complained bitterly that psychiatrists were introducing a foreign and disturbing element into criminal law. The issue arose when insanity or mental aberration was pled, especially in such celebrated cases as Guiteau's shooting of President Garfield in 1880 and the Leopold-Loeb "perfect crime" in 1924. Guiteau, an eccentric office-seeker, brought the issue of "moral insanity" before the court as a basis for acquittal, and the Leopold-Loeb murder, which evolved out of a complex neurotic situation, paraded mental dynamics before the public and the court. Both trials were milestones in forensic psychiatry: The Guiteau affair scuttled the "moral insanity" plea as a viable defense, but the Leopold-Loeb case opened the way for detailed analysis of homicide in murder trials.

I remember that during my second medical year at the University of Cincinnati rumors trickled down from Chicago that homosexuality and crime bore a shadowy relationship to each other. The trial stimulated enormous interest and considerable heat among a startled public. Clarence Darrow, the famous humanitarian lawyer for the defense, consulted Bernard Glueck, William A. White, and William Healy, all psychiatrists, who testified to Leopold's inferiority-superiority complex, his glandular imbalance, and the intellectual super-*mensch* grandiosity that afflicted both defendants. Darrow, who tried the case before a judge without a jury, sought to reduce the sentence from death to life imprisonment on the basis of "diseased motivation."[4] His experts spoke of "split personality," "emotional flatness," and other foreign-sounding concepts. Under Darrow's direction, dynamic psychiatry was introduced into the criminal court. There were, of course, opposing experts, Drs. Patrick and Singer of Chicago, both competent men who disregarded the complex emotional factors that Darrow emphasized and contented themselves with the conclusion that the defendants were sane. After a tense and prolonged trial, Darrow won his plea for mitigation of the death sentence. The outraged public decided that "money talks"; that only the sons of the wealthy could afford such psychiatric luxury. At the time, my fellow students and myself, immersed in pathology, biochemistry, and bacteriology, took little note of this epoch-making event.

However, Darrow's defense, which utilized the testimony of his experts, assisted by Drs. Bowman and Hulbert who had developed the background of the case, was not lost on others. Leaders in the field insisted that "the psychiatrist's chief concern is with understanding and evaluating social and individual factors entering into failure in human life adaptation. . . . Crime is a failure in adaptation."[5] These words issued from a report made in 1926 under the leadership of Karl Menninger, the chairman of the American Psychiatric Association's Committee on Legal Aspects of Psychiatry. It was an impressive document, virtually a white paper that consisted of twenty-two sections: "Criminal behavior and characterologic aberrancies can be scientifically studied, interpreted and controlled. . . . Radical changes must be made in penal practice." The report covered more than the insanity plea; it spoke for a more intimate relationship between law and psychiatry and for effective preventative measures through mental hygiene techniques to combat the "maladaption" called crime. Leaders in the legal profession responded. In 1930 the National Commission on Law Observance and Law Enforcement (the Wickersham Commission), meeting with an American Bar Association committee on which Winfred Overholser was a member, recommended that "the larger courts [should] be encouraged to establish their own psychiatric clinics . . . so each court may have psychiatric services."[6] Until then the county criminal court of New York utilized the services of the Tombs physician, Perry Lichtenstein, an on-the-job trained psychiatrist, and politically connected lunacy commissioners who were appointed by judges. Opposing the haphazard appointments of medicolegal experts, the New York Bar Association and the Forensic Psychiatry Committee of the American Psychiatric Association joined with the New York Society for Medical Jurisprudence to "pool [the] interest and opinions" of the two fields.[7]

As Gregory Zilboorg put it, these were the "golden years of awakening in the field of psychiatric criminal jurisprudence."[8] At a 1934 meeting of the New York Academy of Medicine's section on neurology and psychiatry, Bernard Glueck, who, according to Zilboorg, "represented the advance guard of psychiatry," insisted that "the only hopeful approach to the problem of criminal conduct lies in the application of a scientific individualized [treatment] . . . in place of . . . the mechanical procedure that characterized the legal approach."[9]

The polite coolness between the two disciplines began to thaw in the early 1930s. Some years earlier, in 1921, the Briggs Law had been passed in Massachusetts. It called for the psychiatric examination of all offenders charged with capital crimes or felons with prior convictions for felonies. In this advance, Winfred Overholser had been an effective agent. While rhetoric at medicolegal meetings joined the disciplines in amity, residues of contention between law and medicine still made their appearance in the journals. Psychiatrists like John Kindred complained of the "almost fetichistic workshop of legal criteria of criminal responsibility,"[10] and lawyers reminded psychiatrists that they cannot deal with moral questions (criminal responsibility) ". . . without seeming to invalidate its claim of being a science, not a theology."[11] The criticism, however, did not deter institutional workers from intensively examining convicted offenders. James McCartney of the Elmira Reformatory concluded after conducting psychiatric examinations of the inmates in 1934 that "[they should] be dealt with as mentally sick individuals, who because of some physical, social, intellectual or mental handicap have been adjudged antisocial."[12] In relatively isolated instances, men like the indefatigable Ben Karpman of Saint Elizabeths Hospital in Washington, D.C., persevered in their efforts to understand the individual criminal. In 1933 Karpman published a book of 1,042 pages that painstakingly detailed five criminal cases, their histories and crimes.[13]

As one of Stekel's students, Karpman joined the psychoanalytic movement of the Washington group early in his career, but he soon lost favor with the leaders of the American Psychoanalytic Association, probably because of his approval of Stekel's insistence on the active approach to "leave free scope for the analyst's intuition."[14] Nevertheless, Karpman's studies of psychopathic and sexual criminals at Saint Elizabeths is among the earliest infusion of analytic thinking into the criminal area. His last book, the *Sexual Offender and His Offenses* (1954), which his publishers called "the legitimate inheritor of Krafft-Ebing's *Psychopathia Sexualis*," although somewhat journalistic in tone, constituted an honest effort in this area of criminology. Some regarded Karpman as an eccentric, slightly pathetic figure as he honed down year after year on the psychopathic individual. At one of the American Psychiatric Association meetings in Chicago, Illinois, in about 1936, he pleaded with me to one day write a history of criminologic psychiatry, which was then of interest to a relative few in the profession.

ASSAY INTO CRIMINOLOGY

My entry into criminologic psychiatry was occasioned by two unanticipated circumstances. One was the discovery of a toxic psychosis due to marihuana smoking, which led to an incursion into the criminology of drug usage; the other was an administrative change at Bellevue. These events, initially unrelated, resulted in the pathway to forensic psychiatry.

One day in 1933, two men who had smoked a reefer or two in Harlem were brought into Bellevue Hospital complaining of peculiar feelings: "My head was growing bigger," one said. The other reported, "My head felt unnaturally big, about twice normal size. My arms and legs felt big too." Through his excitement the patient related: "I thought, 'Now I'm going crazy, going to die' . . . I never thought so fast in my life." Within the year eleven cases of Negroes, Caucasians, and Puerto Ricans, were admitted with bizarre complaints after smoking a "funny" cigarette: "It was like heaven, green grass moving . . . My body felt distorted, like in a Coney Island mirror . . . I felt elated in the subway; everybody was my friend . . . I heard a sound like a current . . . the lights red, yellow, blue, green, all moved."

The bizarre symptoms resembled neither schizophrenia nor alcoholic psychosis. Mentioning these odd complaints to Professor Schilder, he remarked: "In Europe, mescaline by German experimenters produced all sorts of distorted fragmentation—visual, touch, auditory." In the meanwhile, scare articles were appearing in the press—"Loco Weed, Breeder of Madness and Crime," "Marihuana as Developer of Criminals." The public prosecutor in New Orleans reported that slightly "less than half of the murders" were by marihuana addicts. Schilder's hint led me to examine the literature on marihuana, which demonstrated that hashish had a long and dishonorable history in the Middle East that was part mythical, part clinical and that *cannabis sativa,* the effective drug in "Indian Weed," caused the peculiar symptoms noted in our cases.[15]

The first group of eleven cases reported in the *Journal of the American Medical Association* in 1934 fell into three groups—acute intoxications lasting two or three days; toxic psychoses lasting several weeks; and toxic psychoses merging into schizophrenic reactions lasting months.[16] More alarming than these symptoms was the reputed tendency of reefers to induce criminal violence. Although the clinical picture of marihuana psychosis was identifiable, the criminal aspect seemed minimal. Scrutiny of 16,000 criminal offenders examined at the court of general sessions in New York County from 1932 to 1937 disclosed only 200 who were marihuana users. Of this group, 21 were convicted of offenses other than drug usage or sale, and only 1 of these was involved with homicide. In spite of these facts, others thought otherwise. All sorts of heinous crimes were imputed to the drug, and "Killer Drug Marihuana" became pablum for journalists. I was invited to a conference convened by the Treasury Department, through Commissioner Harry J. Anslinger, in Washington, D.C., preparatory to framing legislation to limit drug usage. After much discussion a bill, the Marihuana Tax Act, was presented to the Congress and passed in 1937. The use of the drug without medical backing became illegal.

By 1939, thirty-one cases of marihuana psychosis had been collected, which established the clinical syndrome.[17] The conclusion reached in my report concerning its addictive quality stated that marihuana use was a "sensual, hedonistic" habit but not a true addiction. The aura of the demimonde, however, clung to marihuana smoking: Its reported use in Harlem among musicians and the sense of strangeness of a drugged cigarette remained subtly tied to crime and the underworld. Because the report came from the court of general sessions, the omnipresent Mayor Fiorello La Guardia, his pulse on everything in New York from fires to Tammany Hall, called me to his office. The mayor asked if there was a justification for further study of marihuana and crime from a psychiatric point of view. Before I could answer, he opined that what those destined to be criminals needed was "more pasta and less psychiatry." However, he appointed a commission headed by Karl Bowman, the director of the Bellevue Psychiatric Hospital, and a distinguished group of New York pharmacologists, sociologists, psychologists, and psychiatrists, who rendered a long report, affirming that marihuana was not truly addictive and might even have some therapeutic possibilities.[18] There the subject rested until after World War II when marihuana smoking moved from endemic use to a subcultural fad and finally to a national preoccupation.

The second circumstance that catapulted me into the forensic world arose from a Bellevue episode. The staff of Bellevue Psychiatric Hospital, which was young, articulate, and liberal, had been inspired by the political developments in Germany, Italy, and Spain and had developed strong convictions against the oncoming spirit of fascism in the early 1930s. New York, among other centers of liberalism, had taken the League Against War and Fascism to its bosom, particularly when Americans enlisted in the Lincoln Brigade to battle alongside the Loyalist troops in Spain against Generalissimo Franco. Sensitivity toward the rise of fascism joined a generalized rebelliousness toward authority and emerged as displaced anger at our director. Early complaints against Gregory and his assistants flared as the staff demanded that the director of the service be ousted. Almost overnight, residents, junior physicians, and psychologists grouped together against Dr. Gregory's administrative oppression. Charges and countercharges flew, reaching the public ear. Clandestine meetings were held, and explanations that Gregory, who was a physically small man, overcompensated by acting the part of a martinet served as rationalizations. A kind of minor mass hysteria developed that was underlaid with adolescent game playing. The staff called him a "wily Armenian," a sobriquet indicating their defensiveness. Outside the hospital, the reactions to this palace rebellion were vigorous. In 1934 the new commissioner of hospitals in New York City, Dr. S. S. Goldwater, a world renowned hospital administrator and consultant, asked for Gregory's resignation.

The New York press reported that Commissioner Goldwater had "invited complaints from Dr. Gregory's subordinates," and Dr. Goldwater, the director of Mount Sinai Hospital during my service there, had called me about the situation at Bellevue, inquiring about the controversy. The staff complained of Gregory's methods, his tyrannical treatment, his lack of regard for the sensitivities of junior physicians, and his stern demeanor. After several weeks of turmoil, Goldwater forced Gregory's resignation. The reaction of the psychiatric establishment outside the hospital was immediate and vigorous. Comments in the *American Journal of Psychiatry* decried Gregory's dismissal and stated that it was based on "flimsy charges . . . innuendos . . . without consideration of the facts and merits of the situation."[19] Frederick Parsons eulogized Gregory after his death as one who "had to be autocratic [with] questions that could not be timidly dealt with. . . . One who had a razor sharp mind . . . [was] forceful, wise and humane."[20] In time, Karl M. Bowman was appointed director, and with this move, the tempest at Bellevue subsided.

The relevance of this uprising to my forensic career rests on my assignment to the psychiatric clinic of the court of general sessions in 1935. I was put in charge of it when Carter Colbert, the unobtrusive acting director at Bellevue during the interregnum occasioned by the Gregory affair, asked me in an offhand manner if I would like a new career in medicolegal work. I assented and the following six years provided a vista of the possibilities and perplexities of forensic psychiatry.

The New York Court Clinic

The court of general sessions, now known as the Criminal Court of New York County, had a long history that reached back to Revolutionary days. Criminal problems plagued judges then as

now, but the notion of psychiatric study in place of imprisonment
was nonexistent. The flavor of the judicial handling of sexual
crimes, for instance, can be gleaned from a case report of 1807.[21]
A schoolmaster, indicted for "gross indecency toward certain
young females," appeared before the court facing evidence that he
had palpated the buttocks and genitals of the young students
as they stood beside his desk reciting their lessons. The court halted
the prosecuting attorney's recital because it was "unwilling to stain
the pages" with further description of the offender's actions. The
judge "would not hear details so disgusting."

The court clinic was the brainchild of Dr. Gregory. Until its
establishment, the psychiatric examinations conducted by Perry
Lictenstein and the casually appointed lunacy commissions were
related to insanity pleas, and the prisoners were examined either
on the prison ward at Bellevue or in the Tombs Jail. The notion
of investigating the psychodynamics and personality of the criminal
represented a gigantic step forward for psychiatry. It meant an
opening up of the dynamics of noninsane offenders. With this aim
in view, the inception of the clinic followed careful planning by
a group of prominent New York psychiatrists and penologists
with the concurrence of Mayor Jimmy Walker and Dr. William
Greef, the commissioner of health. The clinic was housed on the
floor of the old court building on a level with the famous Bridge
of Sighs. Prisoners awaiting sentence were escorted by heavy-
booted deputy sheriffs from the ancient Tombs Jail to the clinic,
which was manned by psychiatrists of the Bellevue staff. The clinic's
mission was to examine every convicted felon in order to assist
the probation department, which was under Irving Halpern,
chief probation officer, in formulating recommendations to the
judges. The primary task was to establish beyond the presence
or absence of psychosis, the mental level and personality structure
of the criminals who had been convicted of felonies in New York
County.

Two psychiatrists, a clinical psychologist, and secretarial workers
comprised the staff, which examined approximately 2,500 convicted
offenders each year. The infrequent finding of psychotic individuals among the criminal population that passed through the
court had been anticipated by Gregory.[22] With the assistance of

Frederick Wertham, Nathaniel Ross, and Benjamin Apfelberg, he had developed a classification of personality types, ranging from emotionally unstable types through immature, suggestible individuals to outright psychopaths and professional criminals. Although the clinic handled secondary matters—assistance to probation officers in evaluating prospective probationers, pretrial examinations for the judges, and observations of offenders at trial—its main mission was an in-depth personality analysis of a typical criminal population. The analysis of predominant personality traits was expected to permit individual psychiatric treatment of selected cases or at least to make the handling of probationers more perceptive.

The establishment of the clinic was widely hailed as a great advance in criminology. During my eight years with the clinic (it is still active forty-nine years later), thousands of major offenders were examined, analyzed, and pigeonholed, according to their impulses, motivations, personality quirks, and psychopathology. The judges of the court of general sessions agreed in principle that individual attention to criminals was due. They also agreed that "the judge in the past did not, in imposing sentence, regard his act as related in any way to subsequent treatment or the fate of the defendant." The author of this statement, Judge Cornelius F. Collins, pointed out in his lecture before the New York County Bar Association in 1933 that the investigation of the offender's background by the probation department and the clinic reports concerning "*general* mental capacity in the degree that it falls short of 'normal' . . . was a service few courts in this country can boast of."[23] To fill out this ambitious program, there were lectures to probation officers and social workers, which were arranged by Irving Halpern, chief probation officer, and given by prominent neurologists and psychiatrists, including clinic staff members.

In addition to the diagnostic work, the challenge of offering therapy to New York's most accomplished and lesser criminals appealed to me. Here was an opportunity to utilize dynamic understanding of misbehavior in a meaningful area. Arrangements with the chief probation officer and the presiding judge, Cornelius Collins, to treat a few probationers were readily made. Those selected for this advanced idea came after clinic hours through the clanging iron gates to our dingy offices. The setting was anything but favorable: the probationer lay on a hospital stretcher; I sat behind him in a shabby room with bars on the windows. I started bravely and encouraged the probationer to associate freely. The first case, a well-educated man convicted of larceny, who had been a law clerk for a U.S. Supreme Court justice, talked spontaneously, but I had difficulty in relating his conversations to the crime and its motivation. The second case, a middle-aged man convicted of sexually molesting a Western Union messenger boy was more revealing. His inferiority feelings, lack of sexual prowess with women, and general low self-esteem, could be traced to the crime. I felt that the patient, who was relieved of his anxiety by his confession, was probably helped by the therapeutic experience. The third was a young burglar whose crime occurred in an alcoholic fugue state, during which he stole a woman's clothing and property. We were able to uncover some mechanisms of unconscious rivalry with females. The goal of the treatment was to transform the diagnosed psychopathy or criminosis into a neurosis and then to apply a psychoanalytic approach.

Difficulties presented themselves: Many probationers preferred to "do my time in prison" than to be offered probation with its constant surveillance. Others, and this included some of the probation officers, felt that "treatment of crime, which everybody knows has nothing to do with mental illness," could only be attempted by a "nervy" psychiatrist. Probationers could not conceive that the ordinarily hostile, vindictive outside world could have changed its attitude toward criminals. Layers of distrust and veiled anger needed to be removed before psychologizing could be attempted.[24] The subjects were convinced that anyone connected with the courts would be tainted with the desire to inflict subtle psychological torture or had been assigned by a cunning district attorney who wished to ferret out information about New York's underworld. Attempts to befriend prisoners and to win their support for the notion of treatment met with amused resistance. I tried to make the atmosphere informal by playing cards with the offenders on occasion and by convincing our clerk, a former vaudevillian, to lead the men in tap dancing, but it was all to no avail. The treatment attempt had to be abandoned. It was not until the late 1940s that another attempt was made, when Melitta Schmeideberg, head of the Association for Psychiatric Treatment of Offenders, opened her clinic in New York. She was followed by Ralph Banay's Brooklyn Association for the Rehabilitation of Offenders.

The main work of the clinic focused on the pathology of crime and the psychopathology of criminals. The life and miscreancy of the various criminals that passed through our hands rivaled the most imaginative detective story. The search for motivation, conscious and unconscious, among murderers, sex offenders, robbers, burglars, embezzlers, pickpockets, and petty thieves, was amply rewarded. For example, the psychosexual aspect of the swindler's personality, which was worked out with Sylvan Keiser,[25] and the dynamic factors in homicide[26] seemed proof positive that criminal impulses came from the id. But when Karl Bowman discussed our paper, "The Psychology of the Swindler," delivered at the 1937 meeting of the American Psychiatric Association in Pittsburgh, he diplomatically commented that "the attempt to utilize orthodox formulations . . . in our bewildered state as to the cause of a crime . . . depends on audience attitudes towards psychoanalysis."[27]

For all our theorizing, it soon became obvious that most convicted offenders rejected the idea of acknowledging psychological conflicts within themselves. The professional criminal rested secure behind his case-hardened attitude. Lepke Buchalter, who was boss of the Teamsters' Union, which then controlled the lucrative fur and garment industries, as well as a strong-arm man and extortionist, convicted of murder, illustrated this common personality facet. During the psychiatric interviews, he presented an affable front without any signs of psychosis or any personality trait different from the average man in the street. He accepted his antisocial life and subsequent arrests with equanimity as the cost of his periods of affluence, which, although temporary, were considerable. Similarly, Lucky Luciano, "Capo del Capo" of gangsters in New York, presented no evidence of mental aberration or of unconscious conflict, only a tacit recognition of the economic basis of racketeering. While Lucky's defensiveness was firm, his lieutenant, Bellino, said testily at the time of our interview: "You can examine me, Doc, but don't try that psychologic stuff!"

Apart from the professional pickpocket, burglar, and robber whose crimes fitted the socioeconomic mosaic of a metropolis and were without treatable psychological problems, some individuals enmeshed in crime did show neurotic tendencies. Particularly in triangle homicides, the once-in-a-lifetime murderer whose crime climaxed a period of inner tension from fancied or real humiliation (the cuckold reaction) displayed an inordinate sensitivity to sexual inadequacy. Robbers often showed unexpected dependency feelings, which were covered by aggressive fronts. White-collar offenders (notably embezzlers and larcenists) identified with big business and fantasies of omnipotence. A dynamic analytic approach yeilded a great deal of information concerning narcissism, ineffective ego control, early (infantile) dependence reactions, reflections of an unresolved Oedipus complex among sexual criminals, and so on. In general, however, our efforts did not match the high expectations of the Forensic Psychiatry Committee of the American Psychiatric Association. Their published recommendation, "treatment of the petty offender is best done with probationers. . . . [Although] probation is highly developed . . . in only a few does a psychiatric report form part of the material furnished the judge," was only partly fulfilled.[28] Nevertheless, the work continued, and the idea spread.

A CRIMINOLOGIC PSYCHIATRY EVOLVES

Chicago, Boston, Baltimore, and the Detroit traffic court also organized court clinics. Experiences at the New York court clinics shed light on the course and content of criminal careers and provided some insight into acting-out behavior, but *why* unconscious impulses eventuated in criminal action was unknown. My colleagues (Drs. Frederick Wertham, Sylvan Keiser, John Frosch, Nathaniel Ross, and Solomon Machover) and I enjoyed the psychological drama of crime and the opportunity to study various types of offenders. These ranged from Richard Whitney, the Harvard-educated head of the New York Stock Exchange who was convicted of embezzling millions of dollars, to Jimmy

Hines, a Tammany Hall chieftan, convicted of bribery and political chicanery, to Robert Irwin, the Easter Sunday icepick killer, who slew a popular model, her mother, and a male boarder on Manhattan's fashionable East Side. The case became a cause celèbre in the forensic psychiatry community.

Psychopathology and the issue of legal insanity were involved in the Irwin case. Three commissioners in lunacy had been appointed in 1938—an attorney, a neurologist, and a psychiatrist—to render an opinion as to Irwin's capacity to stand trial. The commissioners attempted to examine the accused in his Tombs cell. Because he was considered dangerous (he had made a lunge at me in the clinic office and was regarded as unmanageable), the commissioners stood outside his cell, calling on him to answer. Irwin said nothing. After several attempts, always with the same results, they withdrew and fashioned a report that pronounced Irwin legally sane.[29] The long history of Irwin's psychosis, including his attempt at self-mutilation by castration presumably to enhance his artistic vision, had been studied intensively by Wertham but was discarded by the commission in their report to the court.[30] Wertham in fact developed his concept of "catathymic crisis" in a psychotic setting from the explosiveness Irwin had displayed in the murders. The commission's decision was greeted with dismay in the forensic community. Winfred Overholser, writing from Saint Elizabeths Hospital, denounced the lunacy commission system as too legalistic.[31] He recommended using only those psychiatrists certified by the American Board of Psychiatry and Neurology to make forensic psychiatric examinations of the accused. Probably because of the furor, the certificate of "Commissioner in Lunacy" was abolished in New York soon after.

Meanwhile social scientists were engaged in trying to explain criminality in other than psychopathological terms. Clifford Shaw, a sociologist in Chicago, Illinois, had published his study of juvenile delinquency, which focused on social, that is neighborhood, influences. The Gluecks in Boston analyzed the careers of delinquent boys in respect to personality structure and social environment. For psychiatrists the sociology of crime appeared to be secondary; most medical efforts were expended on the individual, his drives and personality. At times this specificity became controversial. Louis Berman, for example, insisted in the 1930s that endocrine imbalance was the major cause of crime. But his book, *Glands Regulating Personality,*[32] which appeared in 1921, and the more positive *The New Criminology*[33] by Max Schlapp and Edward Smith, which appeared in 1928, were soon discredited. For penologists in prison practice and psychiatrists in court, the outstanding puzzle was the recidivist, the chronic criminal for whom no rehabilitation or treatment effort seemed effective. Here was a fertile field for dynamic study. the antisocial type of psychopathic personality became a formidable quarry for psychological pursuit.

The psychopathic concept, of course, included more than antisocial activity. Sexual deviates were also marked as "psychopaths," that is, as individuals with an unchanging personality bent. Hence it followed that sexual psychopathy engaged the interests of a few analysts. A. A. Brill, for example, wrote on necrophilia.[34] Robert Lindner described the hypoanalysis of a recidivist burglar in the federal penitentiary in Lewisburg, Pennsylvania, whose character formation. Lindner believed, was influenced by witnessing parental intercourse at the age of six months! Lindner's book, *Rebel Without A Cause* became a best-seller and was converted into a motion picture. In it he made the valid point that "the psychopath is a rebel without a cause . . . a prolongation of infantile patterns . . . into the stage of physiological adultism."[35] Psychosexual elements in the development of a psychopath were further detailed by Arthur Foxe, an imaginative psychiatrist whose analysis of a sodomist, among others, at the Dannemora State Hospital in New York led to his notion that crime represented a specific neurosis, a "criminosis."[36] At the time this designation seemed quite apt, but it was not generally adopted. Various crimes, such as kleptomania, were analyzed by Fritz Wittels.[37] And Edmund Bergler, a New York psychoanalyst, invoking Freud's "criminal out of a sense of guilt" theory formulated his "mechanism of orality" theory, which postulated that the criminal (and neurotic) wished masochistically to be caught.[38]

Behind this intensive effort to understand unconscious influences in criminal activity was the trenchant 1931 work of Franz Alexander and Hugo Staub, *The Criminal, the Judge and the Public,* which forcefully introduced American psychiatrists to psychoanalytic insights regarding crime and the legal process.[39] Written in Berlin, where Alexander was an active member of the Berlin Psychoanalytic Association and Staub was a promiment jurist with analytic training, its translation and publication coincided with Alexander's arrival in America to head the Chicago Psychoanalytic Insititute. His elucidation of the neurotic character, which was closely identified with the psychopathic personality, placed him in the front rank of American analysts interested in criminology. Staub, on the other hand, unable to practice criminal law, carried a few patients as a lay analyst but was generally disheartened by the American reaction to his and Alexander's advanced ideas of criminal psychodynamics. On a visit to our court clinic in New York, he recounted his trip to Los Angeles, where he hoped to set up a therapeutic center for offenders. It had come to naught. "California," he said wistfully, "is no El Dorado."

The few psychiatrists involved in forensic and institutional psychiatry continued their studies of the emotional background for crime. A fairly small group, they believed that criminal activity rested on an undoubted neurotic (or psychopathic) core. For this reason, they believed that offenders should be amenable to intensive psychotherapy. But, as experience showed, successful treatment of a recidivist was another matter. As Oberndorf put it, "The discoveries of psychoanalysis are perhaps more valuable in understanding the drives of most criminals than in curing them."[40]

In spite of the different conceptualizations of the psychopathic problem, most workers agreed that the crux of criminal action was somehow related to the mental structure of the psychopath. If that enigma could be solved, we thought, we would know how criminals develop and what could be done about them. Whether inborn or acquired, whether laid down in the brain structure or developed as habitual behavior, the psychopath, in Seymour Halleck's words, "emerged as an important link to the understanding of criminal behavior."[41]

Psychopathic behavior in other areas continued to intrigue thoughtful workers. The character defects, narcissistic personalities in conflict with social customs—social psychopaths, so to speak—met in analytic practice were subject to scrutiny by Phyllis Greenacre, an outstanding New York psychoanalyst. She pointed

to the unconscious effect of family constellations in the development of such persons, especially the influence of a rigid, distant
father and a weak submissive mother.[42] A more generalized
attack on the psychopathic concept was launched by Hervey
Cleckley, who regarded psychopathy as a "genuine and definite
psychiatric disease" that incapacitated the individual socially
"no less than well recognized psychoses."[43] Cleckley, a Rhodes
scholar, urbane Georgian, and fellow member of the Group for
Advancement of Psychiatry in the early post-World War II days,
considered the condition a "psychosis which psychiatry refuses to
face." His book, *The Mask of Sanity*, was highly respected by
many clinicians but did not satisfy analytic efforts to understand
the genesis of the psychopathic personality.

The closer one came to the essence of psychopathy, the more
obscure it became. European authorities were equally at sea.
British psychiatrists followed an older model, stressing distortion
in the "moral sense," that is, "defective control over certain . . .
instinctive desires."[44] The Germans, exemplified by Eugen Kahn,
who was then at Yale University, defined the psychopathic personality as "those . . . [who] are characterized by quantitative
peculiarities in the impulse, temperament or character strata."[45]
He followed the earlier ideas of "constitutional inadequacy" in
slightly different terms: "causally conditioned by biologically rooted
deviations." Americans, for example G. E. Partridge, coining the
term "sociopath," accented the poor social adjustment of the
psychopath: "a persistent behavior pattern in which there is usually
excessive demands."[46]

The capstone of Karpman's three decades of study of psychopaths, published in 1948 under the title of *The Myth of the Psychopathic Personality* divided the symptomatic (neurotic) group from
the idiopathic, or basic, group for which he coined the term
anethopathic.[47] The symptomatic type in reality was a hard-
shelled neurotic whose defense made him appear calloused,
conscienceless, and antisocial. The idiopathic group constituted a
"specific mental disease . . . [in which] personality organization
had a virtual absence of any redeeming social reaction: conscience,
guilt, binding and generous emotions." In this sense Karpman
came close to Cleckley's description of the psychopath as one
suffering from "semantic dementia." My own work with anti-

social individuals led to a different concept. I came to believe that such persons were unconsciously (automatically) reacting to society's distrust and hatred of them by acting as expected, as society's enemies. It was as if the emotionally toned accusations—"constitutionally inferior," "psychopathic inadequate," and the like—thrown at them by generations of psychiatrists expressing their own and society's frustrations, came back like a boomerang with redoubled, or criminal force.[48]

Even brain wave studies did not shed unequivocal light on the constitution of the psychopath.[49] While the coterie of psychiatrists who were interested in unravelling this problem continued their hypotheses, new problems arose as the drug addict and sexual deviate groups were included among the psychopathic personality diagnoses. The sexual psychopath group was especially singled out by the various state legislatures in the face of an alarming increase in sex crimes; for example, the sexual psychopathic laws of Illinois in 1938, Michigan in 1939, and California also in 1939. The interest in these problems continued to grow into the 1940s and 1950s, following the pronouncement of the Forensic Committee of the American Psychiatric Association, which included William A. White, Bernard Glueck, V. C. Branham, and Winfred Overholser, that "crime has become the foremost topic of interest in this nation. . . . Psychiatry on account of its peculiar approach to problems of crime . . . plays a very important [role]."[50] A few voices advised caution in the expressed enthusiasm for psychiatric criminology; thus Menas Gregory once commented in this regard, "Psychiatry might be over-sold."[51]

The puzzle had not yet been solved. Clearly, psychological formulations did not exactly match the varieties of social maladaptations encountered. I thought that perhaps a deeper understanding of the individual psyche, an indepth plumbing of human relations, might shed light on the intricate world of the criminal. Psychoanalysis as a personal experience promised some answers.

NOTES

1. Charles Goring, *The English Convict* (London: H. M. Stationery Office, 1913), p. 369.

2. Carl Murchison, *Criminal Intelligence* (Worcester, Mass.: Clark University Press, 1928), p. 57.

3. Donald J. West and Alexander Walk, eds., *Daniel McNaughton, His Trial and the Aftermath* (England: Headley Bros., Gaskell Books, 1977), p. 9.

4. Irving Stone, *Clarence Darrow for the Defense* (Garden City, N.Y.: Doubleday & Co., 1941), pp. 405-10.

5. Karl Menninger, "Psychiatry in Relation to Crime," in *A Psychiatrist's World*, ed. Bernard H. Hill (New York: Viking Press, 1959), p. 729.

6. "Comments," *American Journal of Psychiatry* 11 (September 1931): 377.

7. "Committee Report: December 1933," *American Journal of Psychiatry* 91 (September 1934): 422.

8. Gregory Zilboorg, "Legal Aspects of Psychiatry," in *One Hundred Years of American Psychiatry*, ed. J. K. Hall (New York: Columbia University Press, 1944), p. 576.

9. Proceedings of the New York Neurological Society, "Psychiatry and the Criminal Law," *Journal of Nervous and Mental Disease* 2 (February 1935): 192-212.

10. John J. Kindred, "Insanity in Its Medico-legal Relations to Some Notable Criminal and Civil Cases," *American Journal of Psychiatry* 91 (July 1934): 137.

11. Edward De Grazia, "The Distinction of Being Mad," *University of Chicago Law Review* 22 (1945-55): 339.

12. James L. McCartney, "An Intensive Psychiatric Study of Prisoners in the Receiving Routine in the Classification Clinic Elmira Reformatory," *American Journal of Psychiatry* 90 (May 1934): 1184.

13. Ben Karpman, *Case Studies in the Psychopathology of Crime*, 2 vols. (Washington, D. C.: Mineoform Press, 1933; rpt. ed., New York: Mental Science Publ. Co., 1939).

14. Donald L. Burnham, "Orthodoxy and Eclecticism in Pschoanalysis, The Washington-Baltimore Experience," in *American Psychoanalysis*, ed. Jacques Quen and Eric Carlson (New York: Brunner Mazel, 1978), p. 97.

15. Lester Greenspann, *Marihuana Reconsidered* (Cambridge, Mass.: Harvard University Press, 1971), chap. 4, p. 55 et seq.

16. Walter Bromberg, "Marihuana Intoxication: A Clinical Study of Cannabis Sativa Intoxication," *American Journal of Psychiatry* 91 (September 1934): 303-30.

17. Walter Bromberg, "Marihuana, a Psychiatric Study," *Journal of the American Medical Association* 13 (July 1939): 4.

18. "Mayor's Committee on Marihuana, Charles B. Wallace, M.D.,

Chairman," in *The Marijuana Papers,* ed. D. Solomon (Indianapolis: Bobbs-Merrill Co., 1966), p. 233 et seq.

19. "Comment," *American Journal of Psychiatry* 91 (November 1934): 707.

20. Frederick W. Parsons, "In Memoriam, Menas S. Gregory," *American Journal of Psychiatry* 98 (January 1942): 631.

21. People v. W.W. Jenner, Court of General Sessions of the Peace (1816).

22. Walter Bromberg and Charles B. Thompson, "The Relation of Psychosis, Mental Defect and Personality Types to Crime," *Journal of Criminal Law and Criminology* 28 (May-June 1937): 70-89.

23. Cornelius F. Collins, "Treatment of Criminals in the Court of General Sessions of the County of New York," *Journal of Criminal Law and Criminology* 24 no. 4 (November-December 1933): 700.

24. Walter Bromberg, "Psychotherapy in a Court Clinic," *American Journal of Orthopsychiatry* 11 (October 1941): 770-74.

25. Walter Bromberg and Sylvan Keiser, "The Psychology of the Swindler," *American Journal of Psychiatry* 94 no. 6 (May 1938): 1441-58.

26. Walter Bromberg, *The Mold of Murder, A Psychiatric Study of Homicide* (New York: Grune & Stratton, 1961).

27. K. Bowman, "Discussion of 'The Psychology of the Swindler,'" *American Journal of Psychiatry* 94 (May 1938): 1456-58.

28. "Comment," *American Journal of Psychiatry* 92 (September 1936): 460.

29. "Report of Commissioners in Lunacy: People vs. Irwin," *American Journal of Psychiatry* 95 (July 1938): 219-25.

30. Frederick Wertham, *The Show of Violence* (Garden City, N. Y.: Doubleday & Co., 1949) p. 120.

31. Winfred Overholser, Letter to the Editor, *American Journal of Psychiatry* 95 (November 1938): 733.

32. Louis Berman, *The Glands Regulating Personality* (New York: Macmillan, 1921).

33. Max G. Schlapp and Edward H. Smith, *The New Criminology* (New York: Boni and Liveright, 1928).

34. A. A. Brill, "Necrophilia," *Journal of Criminal Psychopathology* 2 (April 1941): 433-43, and 3 (July 1941): 50-72.

35. Robert Lindner, *Rebel Without a Cause: The Hypoanalysis of a Criminal Psychopath* (New York: Grune & Stratton, 1944), p. 2.

36. Arthur Foxe, *Crime and Sexual Development* (Glens Falls, N. Y.: The Monograph Editor, 1936).

37. Fritz Wittels, "Kleptomania and Other Psychopathic Crimes,"

Journal of Criminal Psychopathology 4 (October 1943): 205.

38. Edmund Bergler, "The Mechanism of Oral-Neurosis and Criminosis," in *Handbook of Correctional Psychology,* ed. R. Lindner and R. V. Seliger (New York: Philosophic Library, 1947), pp. 611-31.

39. Franz Alexander and Hugo Staub, *The Criminal, the Judge, and the Public,* trans. Gregory Zilboorg (New York: Macmillan Co., 1931).

40. Clarence Oberndorf, "Sidelights on Criminality From Psychoanalytic Practice," in *Handbook of Correctional Psychology,* p. 678.

41. Seymour Halleck, "American Psychiatry and the Criminal, A Historical Review," *American Journal of Psychiatry* 121 (March 1965) suppl. 1.

42. Phyllis Greenacre, "Conscience in the Psychopath," *American Journal of Orthopsychiatry* 15 (July 1945): 495-509.

43. Hervey Cleckley, *The Mask of Sanity* (St. Louis: C. V. Mosby Co., 1941), p. 418.

44. W. Lewis, *A Textbook of Mental Diseases,* 2d ed. (London: Chas. Griffen and Co., 1899).

45. Eugen Kahn, *Psychopathic Personalities,* trans. H. Flanders Dunbar (New Haven: Yale University Press, 1931), pp. 62, 312.

46. G. E. Partridge, "A Study of Fifty Cases of Psychopathic Personality," *American Journal of Psychiatry* 7 (May 1928): 953.

47. Benjamin Karpman, "The Myth of the Psychopathic Personality," *American Journal of Psychiatry* 104 (March 1948): 523-24.

48. Walter Bromberg, "The Treatability of the Psychopath," *American Journal of Psychiatry* 110 (February 1954): 604-8.

49. D. Silverman, "Clinical and E.E.G. Studies of Criminal Psychopaths," *Archives of Neurology and Psychiatry* 50 (1943): 18-33.

50. "Forensic Psychiatry Committee Report," *American Journal of Psychiatry* 11 (September 1931): 823.

51. Menas S. Gregory, "Psychiatry and the Problems of Delinquency," *American Journal of Psychiatry* 101 (January 1935): 773.

6
THE MIDDLE GAME

By the mid-1930s, the psychiatric scene had fanned out to include a wide array of treatment methods and their attendant theories. The number of practicing psychiatrists nationally had increased several fold; correspondingly, the supply of patients mounted. New York lost its position as the Mecca of psychiatry, except for psychoanalysis. The major universities in the East, Midwest, and West had sprouting, or settled, departments of psychiatry. Throughout the nation, especially in the larger cities, mental hygiene ideas had permeated the primary schools and colleges; social services had accepted psychological tenets in their case work; the orthopsychiatric movement had gathered psychiatrists, psychologists, psychiatric social workers, and child guidance personnel—all who dealt with emotional problems—into its capacious arms.

The enthusiasm and driving force behind this increase in psychiatric activity was directly reflected in two diverging areas. One was the trend toward biochemical treatment techniques, the other toward dynamic, interpretive therapy. Both were hailed as "breakthroughs." Therapeutic optimism survived the years of the Great Depression even though a decrease in the funds available for personal and institutional treatment exerted an effect. A nationwide survey of state hospitals by the National Committee for Mental Hygiene between 1930 and 1936 found "drastic budget cuts, cessation of building programs, over-crowding, slowing-up of therapy, [and] fear of regression to custodial care."[1] Yet innovators continued their search for new methods of treatment. Biochemical techniques touched on such diverse areas as experiments with various kinds of narcosis to reduce resistance toward "revealing hidden sources of conflict" in patients,[2] hormone therapy in depressions,[3] and insulin and metrazol shock therapy by Manfred Sakel,[4] and others. The physicochemical methods were tremendously stimulating; the dynamic techniques were no less exciting.

THE SHOCK ERA

Insulin shock, which came to be regarded as a revolution in the management of schizophrenics, followed Sakel's discovery in Vienna of improved behavior and mental clarity among drug addicts subjected to hypoglycemia. On the assumption that these favorable results followed from the chemical changes in the cerebral cell bodies brought about by insulin-induced hypoglycemia, Sakel carried the technique to his schizophrenic patients. The results were spectacular in terms of remissions. The apparent ability of reduced blood sugar to alter brain chemistry provided a degree of scientific sanction to this empirical method.[5] It was introduced to New York by the Bellevue psychiatric service as the result of Joseph Wortis's visit to Sakel's clinic in Vienna. Wortis, a sort of free-roving psychiatric investigator, had worked with Havelock Ellis in England on a grant to study psychosexuality; he also had been given the opportunity to spend several months between 1934 and 1935 in a "learning" analysis with Freud.[6] During this time, Wortis visited the Pötzl Klinic, where Sakel's insulin shock therapy program was in progress. Before bringing the method to Bellevue Hospital, he wrote home about "one of the most remarkable things I had ever seen." Bernard Glueck, founder of Stony Lodge, a private sanatorium in Ossining, New York, also journeyed to Sakel's clinic. Delighted with what he witnessed, he remarked, "I rolled up my sleeves and went to work."[7]

The first reports of shock therapy on schizophrenics were startling. Patients with relatively short histories (a year or less) of illness responded well. At Bellevue, Wortis and his associates commented that the hypoglycemia method was "the best treatment available for schizophrenics."[8] Universal interest was aroused, and soon the journals were filled with reports of experiences with schizophrenics treated by the hypoglycemic method. Patients with recent histories showed marked improvement, 70 percent to 88 percent remissions.[9] For several years enthusiasm ran high; the press lauded the "miracle" cure; and many families burdened with chronically ill sons and daughters clamored for insulin shock treatment. But complications developed, such as irreversible coma, fractures after convulsions, and briefer remissions in chronic cases. The Committee on Public Education, which was headed by the American Psychiatric Association, felt impelled to voice "regret . . . if insulin shock treatment should be a means of holding out a false hope to the families of tens of thousands of sufferers of Dementia Praecox."[10]

For the next two decades, shock treatment—Metrazol, insulin, and electroshock—with modifications and improvements in technique was discussed in literally thousands of papers and monographs.[11] Kalinowsky and Hoch's treatise in 1950 covers much of the early work.[12] My own experience in the 1930s was confined to one attempt to use Metrazol with a depressive patient whom I treated privately. A few treatments seemed to help, but the violence of the major convulsion abruptly following injection of the medication shocked me and my associate.

Metrazol soon gave way to electroconvulsive therapy and its amendments and improvements. From the 1940s on, there was hardly a sanatorium, hospital, or private office, that did not use the method, and there were few practicing psychiatrists (including this one) who did not possess a "buzz" box, the black box in which the electroshock machine was housed. The literature on electroshock grew enormously, and with it, the number of treatments given certain patients escalated from a series of 20 to as high as 200 in some hospitals. A number of schizophrenic and many depressive patients seemed to do well with the treatment. One explanation put forth was the effect of the electric current on the diencephalic centers of the brain. Other observers felt that the improvement followed the psychological shock of annihilation with a "re-establishment of adaptive defensive" mechanisms.[13] Most experimenters agreed that whatever the mechanical effect on the brain cells, "the impending death and rebirth . . . mobilized vital instincts of the patients."[14] In any event, electroshock therapy remained an important agency for shortening depressions and improving reality contact among schizophrenic patients.

SPREAD OF PSYCHOLOGICAL THERAPY

Medical and biochemical methods of treatment primarily concerned sick individuals. However, the neurotic and depressed persons who were presenting themselves in increasing numbers to psychiatrists for help with life's problems asked for less drastic procedures. Even professionals were slightly uneasy in the face of empirical techniques that produced results without clear-cut explanations of how they did so. The rationale for the success of shock treatment could not be established directly; it required a fresh viewpoint and possible laborious research into the intricacies of brain function. Psychoanalysis, although not free from complex and often convoluted theorizing, dealt with feelings and strivings that could be confirmed through free associations, dream analysis, and historical reconstructions. More and more of the profession found themselves in agreement with Fenichel's pronouncement: "There are many ways to treat neuroses, but there is only one way to understand them. . . . There is but one theory to give a scientific explanation of the effectiveness of *all* psychotherapies."[15] Patients and public both appeared to agree that probing the emotions and memories of childhood and untangling the results of these experiences, was the road to mental health.

Mental hygienists who had broached analytic concepts indirectly through child guidance, sex education, or therapy with delinquents laid the foundation for the public acceptance of the psychological approach to emotional problems.[16] A comment in a 1936 issue of *Mental Hygiene* characterized as healthy the "growing interest in mental disorders as a topic of public discussion. . . . No longer is the subject confined to professional and technical journals."[17] It pointed to a series of "highly interesting, understanding, and informative articles" in *Scribner's Magazine, Fortune, Reader's Digest, True Story,* and *Physical Culture* that carried such titles as "Your Chances of Going Insane," "The Nervous Breakdown," and "That Queer Feeling." Elizabeth Adamson's book, *So You're Going to a Psychiatrist,* published in 1936, helped to bridge the gap between the intricacies of analytic theory and the average patient.[18] In fact, the need for psychological insight into one's emotions had become democratized among the American public in the fourth decade of this century and reached even fuller expression after World War II. The rugged individualism of previous generations took a slightly different turn in extolling the importance of an "internal standard . . . of one's measure of worth."[19] This underlay one of the messages of mental hygiene: acknowledgement of an "unconscious mind" that affected conscious behavior and attitudes and the control of which could bring self-realization.

The influence of psychoanalysis in indirectly focusing attention on the importance of self-knowledge cannot be underestimated. A generation later, in the 1960s, Abraham Maslow, invoking a "self-actualization . . . of one's potentialities" concept of humanistic psychology, openly espoused what had been adumbrated by psychoanalytical theory and therapy.[20] The urge to enjoy the mental freedom to shed infantile drawbacks and unburden oneself of repressions appealed to the literate public. It is a fair assumption that this striving to live unhampered by neurotic quirks played a large but silent part in the growth of psychoanalysis in this country. Perhaps this desire represented a forerunner of existentialism, an accent on self-knowledge as a prelude to a better, more rational life, or perhaps it was a return to the older Jamesian accent on the "will" but with a difference.[21]

The aim of psychoanalysis was to free the individual from the repressions and distortions induced by unconscious conflicts, and thus allow him or her to choose his or her aims and aspirations, not simply utilize the will as a matter of self-discipline. As Donald Burnham, a psychoanalyst and historian of psychiatric social-culturism, put it in another context, "perhaps [the] American emphasis on optimism and meliorism contributed" to the acceptance of psychoanalysis as the road to psychological freedom.[22]

While pursuit of the elusive cause of and cure for neurotic afflictions increased in intensity, new approaches evolved. Count Alfred Korzybski, building on the work of Polish mathematicians and physicists, wrote *Science and Sanity,* an exposition of general semantics in relation to mental disease.[23] His basic theory stated that the "actual conditions of life are shaped by *extensional science* (mathematics and physics), while our inner orientation and the structure of language remains intensional."[24] From this standpoint, Count Korzybski stated that we live on a level of abstractions that is not the same as the real (object) world. Semantics, therefore, has brought us to an unsane world through excessive rationalizing. (I must confess that I was unable to read the original, ponderous volume and consulted an outline of his work from an excellent review in the 1934 *Psychoanalytic Quarterly* by Markus Reiner, a philosopher.[25]) According to Korybski's thesis, because of our "excessive rationalizing, our expectations are not fulfilled"; we confuse real objects with semantics, but "a thing is not the same as a word about it." The result, Korzybski claimed, was a "semantic shock" that placed us in an unsane world. The basis of his work called for a philosophic reorientation, a "non-aristotelian logic," which was an interesting proposition but one not readily applicable to clinical or therapeutic work.

Language as the basis of human thinking, however, could not be dismissed so easily. Thinking and language disorders among schizophrenics and organic brain disease patients intrigued investigators. Harry Stack Sullivan pointed out that the peculiarities of schizophrenic speech rested on social and individual insecurity.[26] Norman Cameron found the schizophrenic "scattered" speech to depend on the inability to "restrict, eliminate, [or] focus on the task in hand."[27] Kurt Goldstein, who developed tests to measure cognitive defects in organic brain cases, found schizophrenics to labor under the same difficulties in abstract ideas.[28] Their tendency toward "concretistic thinking" became evident in the Vigotsky sorting test, which was brought here from Russia in 1930 by Jacob Kasanin.[29] Samuel Beck, working with the then new Rorschach test, found through their neologisms and distorted responses that schizophrenics have a "poor apprehension" of the real world.[30] Kasanin, who collated these researches, started his activities on the East Coast in Boston and New York and eventually became director of the psychiatric department of the Mount Zion Hospital in San Francisco. An ebullient personality, much loved by his co-workers, Kasanin did much to stimulate psychoanalytic interest among West Coast psychiatrists and psychiatric social workers.

Still another approach dedicated to displacing the psycho-analytic influence was John Watson's behaviorism.[31] Strictly a development of physiologic psychology and founded on Bechterev's conditioned reflex theories, behaviorism's chief use was in education, but it also impinged on psychotherapy. Although the attempts of Watson and his followers, Clark L. Hull and B. F. Skinner, to replace instinct with conditioning received scientific support from Horsley Gantt in Baltimore and others, it was strongly rejected by the academic majority and by analytically trained psychiatrists. Behaviorism threatened introspection as a psychological instrument and instinct theory as a fundamental to psychoanalysis and thus engendered almost as much heated controversy between 1915 and 1930 as Freudianism. As Kazdin remarked in his *History of Behavior Modification*, "Watson exalted objectivism . . . regarding subjective states as inappropriate topics for scientific study," which justifiably raised the hackles of analysts.[32] However, after World War I, in nonacademic circles behaviorism functioned as an advanced movement that liberated child training from the swaddling clothes of the post-Victorian era. Progressive parents and progressive schools embraced behaviorism; education was altered to accept emotional training as more significant than the "three R's." Nevertheless, psychiatric clinicians continued to bypass Watson's and Skinner's claims until the 1960s, when Joseph Wolpe proposed reconditioning as an effective therapeutic technique.[33]

The Psychiatric Scene

The antipsychological bias of Watson-Skinner behaviorism aided the decreasing antipsychoanalytic feeling. By the mid-1930s the process of denying Freudianism as a part of modern psychiatry had been relegated to a sort of game. When Albert Moll, a German psychiatrist of Freud's generation wrote a book entitled *A Lifetime of Mental Healing* in 1936, Fritz Wittels in the *Psychoanalytic Quarterly* called it "an excellent example of the obsolete wholesale rejection of psychoanalysis."[34] When Moll wrote, "I wish to set myself against the fairy tale that Freud has discovered the subconscious or the unconscious," Wittels said, "The book [Moll's] is psychotherapy on the level of a tabloid column healer." The following year Phyllis Greenacre in a review of Josephine

Jackson's *Guiding Your Life,* a popular mental health exposition, wrote, "The book combines the literary tones of an old-fashioned syndicated health column . . . and mental hygiene recipes."[35] In essence, theoretical and clinical psychoanalysis had reached the position of an accepted addition to psychiatry through a codification of the total mental life of man. By 1938 Franz Alexander in his address, "Psychoanalysis Comes of Age," before the fortieth meeting of the American Psychoanalytic Association indicated the maturity of the dynamic view by calling for a "newer critical appraisal . . . [and the need for] a scientific spirit . . . even quantitative tests of psychodynamic formulations."[36] Although Alexander recognized the "earmarks of our romantic and heroic past" from which he urged analysts to "emancipate" themselves, he counseled a "flexible" approach that would be open to "innovations." In a word, psychoanalysts now were comfortable with their inclusion in the corpus of psychiatry and through the growing field of psychosomatics, into medicine as well.

Even with this consolidation of the expanding theories and techniques concerning mental illness and abnormalities, there still did not exist an identifiable criterion as to whom could be called a bona fide psychiatrist. The solution to this problem came through the efforts of Walter Freeman, a neurologist and neuropathologist at George Washington University. In 1934 he hit upon the happy idea of qualifying specialists under an American Board of Psychiatry and Neurology. Through a group of competent, outstanding specialists, a plan was developed to examine candidates after adequate residency preparation for certification as qualified psychiatrists and/or neurologists. The board's aim was to "separate specialists-in-fact from specialists-in-name." In 1937 I applied and was accepted for the examination at the University of Pennsylvania Hospital. It was a humid day in June when David Impastato of Bellevue, myself, and a few others from the New York area, traveled to Philadelphia under the spell of a mild case of examination anxiety. The examiners promised to be a formidable group. We knew that Adolf Meyer would be among them, and in preparation Impastato and I rehearsed the "ergasias," a term Meyer had developed to replace the more familiar psychiatric phrases. It was an unwieldy concept as Meyer's own definition revealed: "Each ergasia or psychobiological action phase unit implies discriminative and associative, orientative, and constructive functions, and consists of topical . . . and regulative . . . components.''[37] Luckily Meyer examined me only on neuroanatomy, as if already informed of our cramming sessions on the ergasias. Walter Freeman asked for a discussion of multiple sclerosis; Hans Reese of Chicago queried a case of Freidreich's ataxia; Bernard Alpers of Philadelphia demonstrated pneumoencephalographs; and Clarence Cheney presented a schizophrenic patient for discussion. As I recall, the candidates qualified in both neurology and psychiatry. At the end of two humid days, we congratulated each other over a few beers on our expected elevation and went our separate ways.

Nothing spectacular occurred when I achieved my certification in neurology and psychiatry. I had already moved to Lawson Lowrey's office on West Fifty-fourth Street, which brought me into closer contact with the orthopsychiatric group of which Lowrey was a prime mover. The hospital and court work continued; after-hours practice was sluggish. I attempted intensive psychotherapy with a few cases and cared for a few patients in private sanatoria in New York and environs. Private mental hospitals were graded in the attention and comfort they provided patients and in the grounds and appurtenances they offered. A few employed analytic methods, but the majority functioned in a way similar to the state hospitals with less crowding and more amenities. They also introduced insulin shock treatment, electroshock, and milieu therapy. Those families in the New York area with adequate financial backing used the Bloomingdale Hospital in White Plains, the Long Island Home in Amityville, Stony Lodge in Ossining, or West Hill in Riverdale. Smaller places such as Halcyon Rest in Rye (the name carried a certain after-death flavor), the Towne Clinic (primarily for alcoholics and drug addicts) on Central Park West, and Dr. Henry Rogers's ''home'' on Edgcombe Avenue were valuable alternatives to state hospitals for those who were still sensitive to the alleged humiliation of commitment to a public institution.

Meanwhile, the therapeutic horizon had enlarged gradually. Ancillary therapies—occupational, recreational, group sessions— enlivened the boredom of institutional life. In state hospitals these niceties could not always be honored. However, efforts in that direction, the "total push" therapy, which was espoused by Abraham Myerson of Boston, strove to forestall deterioration in schizophrenic patients by such activities as games, personal grooming, exercises, crafts, and so forth.[38] Building on earlier efforts in this direction by W. A. Bryan, superintendent of the Danvers State Hospital in Massachusetts, the "total push" routine enlisted all staff members of the hospital (the therapeutic team) in stimulating the ego of regressed patients to their hospital milieu and, hopefully, to the outside world.[39]

Office practice was another matter. Since potential patients accepted analysis as the royal road to social adjustment, sexual satisfaction, and personality improvement, younger psychiatrists attempted intensive psychotherapy. A couch, a quiet office, and attentive listening seemed to suffice. Seasoned neurologists, picking up some of the phraseology of analysis, listened to their patients with more forebearance and encouraged free associations as they placed their patients "under treatment." One could read Freud's works *in toto* or any of the excellent texts on the subject (Ives Henrick's, Martin Peck's or Lawrence Kubie's) and even place patients on the couch as many nonanalysts did, thus practicing a sort of tamed "wild" analysis. But it was not psychoanalysis. The debate over the necessity of a personal "didactic" analysis, which had raged for years, had long since been settled. The argument that Freud himself had not been analyzed by another was met with an indulgent smile. How could one solve a patient's resistances if one's own had not been analyzed? The counter-argument was unanswerable.

A Psychoanalytic Candidate

My first contact with the analysts at Brill's brownstone home in the West Seventies, close by Central Park, occurred while I was still a resident at Mount Sinai. The meeting was informal with many early members of the New York Psychoanalytic Society present. Dr. Brill presented in his easy manner, discussing his and others' clinical experiences. The atmosphere was relaxed. As Samuel Atkin put it in a later review of the beginnings of analysis in New York, "Students were invited . . . without fixed requirements, as to a learned society."[40] I was, as were we all, charmed by Brill. His open discussion of psychosexuality, the faintly roguish manner with which he spoke to medical or lay audiences, his willingness to talk to anyone who would listen about his early experiences at Burghölzli in Zurich, where he and Jung analyzed their dreams at the breakfast table, diluted any feeling of veneration, even fear, such as I imagined Freud himself would have engendered. Over the years I talked to him, or more accurately listened to him, off-stage, so to speak, at psychiatric meetings. He never paraded his learning or complained of his early struggles, for he was content as a tireless proselytizer to advance the cause of psychoanalysis.

There was an openness about Brill that suggested a friendly physician whose wisdom emerged through stories always with a calculated point. Whatever his manner in a treatment situation, Brill's liveliness outside shone through his humor and humanity. Once at a meeting, he answered a questioner from the audience about sexual deviancy (oral copulation) by the smiling rejoinder: "It's all a matter of taste." His scraggly Van Dyke beard belied his democratic, one might say plebian, leanings. Once he told of saying to a prospective female patient who seemed reluctant to accept analytic treatment: "For a thousand dollars, I can cure you in three months!" At another time, he related his invitation to a seven-day Caribbean cruise, arranged by a philanthropist, to which leaders in philosophy, psychology, political science, and economics were chosen to come up with a definite solution for the world's trouble. "We settled nothing on the cruise" he said.[41] Despite Brill's earthy manner, he was respected by associates and loved by students.

As the Freudian libido theory gave way to the more comprehensive "ego" paradigm, one heard hints that Brill's espousal of earlier libidinal phases was slightly old-fashioned. At the time, my impression, and that of others, was of a courageous man who was comfortable in his position as psychoanalytic seer and interested in every aspect of the field and in everyone who wished to learn. At the 1931 joint meeting of the American Psychiatric Association and the American Psychoanalytic Association in Toronto, Brill presented a psychological study of President

Abraham Lincoln the man, discussing the influence of Lincoln's unconscious anal traits on his depressive affect and mordant humor.[42] This bit of psychohistory about our country's great invoked much discussion at the meeting and some protests by the press. Still, a commentator in the *Psychiatric Quarterly* wrote that "No great harm resulted" from Brill's analysis of Abe Lincoln in absentia.[43]

Brill's influence on such analytic peripheralists as myself was matched by that of Clarence Oberndorf. In 1921 "Oby" became one of the handful of Americans (of whom Adolph Stern was the first) to be analyzed by Freud. Eight years before his analysis, he had organized an outpatient clinic at Mount Sinai in which he used analytic concepts with patients. Later he became the first psychoanalyst to be appointed to a neurological service.[44] Oberndorf represented a different genre than Brill. Soft of speech, a reflection of his South Carolinian background, "Oby" encouraged younger men to share his extensive experience in psychoanalysis.[45] His interest in literature (he had written of Dr. Oliver Wendell Holmes's perception of the unconscious as portrayed in his novels) cast a connoisseurlike glow to his conversation on hospital wards and at meetings.[46] Oby was especially kind to me; he once invited me to his office on Fifty-ninth Street, overlooking Central Park, to suggest that I travel to Zurich to look into a new test developed by one Hermann Rorschach that promised a revelation in probing mental pathology. Unwisely, I declined.

With these experiences a didactic analysis could no longer be forestalled. As a prospective student in training at the New York Psychoanalytic Institute, I had to choose an analyst. The process of seeking out an analyst for an analyzand was little discussed as it was presumed that they were all equally trained to ferret out the nuclear Oedipus complex. On the presumption that the recent flood of émigrés from Vienna and Germany, now under the Hitlerian whiplash, would be closest to the Freudian fountainhead, I approached Fritz Wittels, a genial person with a reputation for literary attainments as well as valid psychoanalytic training. Perhaps the choosing or rejecting of an analyst had to do with one's resistances. In any event, the interview with Wittels progressed easily until he casually mentioned something to the effect: "There are two directions in analysis—heterosexual and homosexual." Without knowing exactly why, I felt his formula was pat and simplistic. Years later, Kardiner in reviewing his experience in Vienna wrote, "In analysis, Freud made a beeline for the Oedipus conflict. His favorite way of resolving this syndrome was in terms of 'unconscious homosexual conflict'."[47]

Recalling Atkin's recommendation of Kardiner as an "intelluctual" type, that is, his analyst, I applied and was accepted as an analyzand. The move stirred a feeling of elation; now, I thought, the bedrock of personality would be reached. As Melitta Schmeideberg said in a discussion of the afterlife of an analytic patient: "[The patient] expects . . . after being fully analyzed [that] he will never have any more difficulties or disappointments in life . . . will develop remarkable intellectual or esthetic powers, perhaps even prove to be a genius . . . be perfectly balanced [and] superhumanly unbiased."[48] In short, Schmeideberg concluded, "The possibilities of analytic therapy are likely to stimulate the ideas of grandeur inherent in all of us."

Kardiner's office, a spacious apartment on Park Avenue, seemed to embody the essence of psychoanalysis. No rush of patients, no telephone. I never saw a patient leaving; I only had the feeling of one having been there recently. The sessions extended to five days a week, and the fee was a considerable item in our family budget but not exorbitant. I reassured myself that Dr. Kardiner was a competent psychiatrist; his work on war neurosis had received wide and favorable reaction. He sat behind the couch enveloped in a blue cloud of smoke and made occasional astute observations, some of which forty-five years later still ring true. Since I had imagined a didactic analysis to be a sort of preceptorship, I was surprised to discover that little direct teaching was done. But some comments bore on future analytic practice, for he remarked one day, "One has to develop one's own technique of analysis."

On the couch, I entered into a detailed history of my family, my sexual life, the trivia of marriage, the clinic, my likes and dislikes, my frustrations and angers. Dreams of which I had, and still have, a constant supply came tumbling out; free associations flowed. The process sounded like an analysis as projected in the textbooks. Beyond that nothing much happened for months except a faint, uneasy feeling that had no direction or object. I remarked to Kardiner that I felt as if I were in a desert and attacked from changing positions by fast-moving, white-robed Bedouins who blended into the sand dunes. My frustration continued: I cried out, "I'd like to meet them face to face." Kardiner said quietly: "That's your unconscious—you'll meet it soon." After eighteen months, Kardiner finally said, "We'll stop for awhile and see how it works out."

Meanwhile, I had become a student-in-training at the New York Psychoanalytic Institute. The easy informality of occasional contacts with Brill, Oberndorf, Philip Lehrman, Dudley Schonfeld, and others gave way to firm student-requirements.[49] They started with a "preparatory analysis," for those candidates possessing an M.D. degree, training in psychiatry at a recognized mental hospital, a "suitable" personality, a pledge of "good faith" not to undertake psychoanalytic work without authorization from the educational committee, and an application form with the enrollment fee of twenty-five dollars. The educational committee made all the decisions concerning "personal suitability," and checked the progress of the preparatory analysis, which they had determined should "not consist of less than three hundred analytic hours."

Kardiner's parting tone at the end of about 275 hours sounded faintly ominous. Soon after, the educational committee requested that I see Dr. Zilboorg, presumably for a review of my suitability.[50] Gregory Zilboorg, in contrast to other analysts I had met or had come to know, was regarded as a flamboyant character. Equipped with a walrus mustache in those clean-shaven days, a scholarly gait, and stoop to match, he was reputed to have been an undersecretary in the Kerensky government early in the 1917 Russian revolution. His analytic training in Vienna and Berlin in conjunction with rather wide scholarship gave his utterances a professorial, if not a downright theatrical coloring. It was reported that he had lectured on the Chautauqua circuit, and the students listening to his remarks at the institute meetings were prone to comment sotto voce, "Next week, East Lynne." Still, one had to balance Zilboorg's pomposity against his research attainments in psychiatric history, his philosophic and forensic papers, and his clinical work at the New York Hospital in White Plains.

On the appointed day, I entered Zilboorg's office, or rather first entered a waiting room graced by a receptionist, then a preinterview room through which a secretary flitted, and finally his consulting chamber. After a few pleasantries he explained that perhaps a second analysis would be in order and suggested Adolph Stern. Just what resistance had been encountered in my case was not clear; I recall thinking that I had been impressed by the notion of "temperament," which Eugen Kahn had discussed in detail but generally was neglected among dynamic psychiatrists as an anachronism of Teutonic philosophic-psychiatry.[51] For some years Kahn, then at Yale University, had promulgated the view that "the way of experiencing [by] various aspects of personality, has . . . the closest affinity to temperament . . . tied to the autonomic, neuro-endocrine system and its centers in the diencephalon."[52] I consoled myself with the reminder that, according to my mother, I had been a precipitate delivery and hence a hyperkinetic type. In any event, resistances had to be overcome.

The second analyst, Adolph Stern, represented a different sort of surrogate father. He had been the first American analyzand of Freud's; I reveled in the fantasy that I would thus become, psychoanalytically speaking, the grandson of the master. But instead of lying on the couch, Stern sat me across from his desk so that we could talk face to face. I later found out that this technique had been developed from his experiences with cases demonstrating narcissistic defenses, which he detailed in his paper, "Psychoanalytic Investigation of and Therapy in the Border Line Group of Neuroses."[53] This notion of character analysis, which was introduced by Wilhelm Reich, a German analyst, focused on the protective "armour" of the patient's ego.[54] His original concept, a major advance, opened the area for psychoanalytic treatment of those cases in whom transference was not easily developed. Unfortunately, Reich, when he came to America, embraced a new concept, "a universal primordial energy . . . BIOENERGY . . . Orgone energy," which deviated so widely from current analytic theory to place him beyond the pale.[55] In commenting on one of his works, *Die Bione* (*Orgone*), Martin

Grotjahn wrote that it would "shock the reader who remembers the time when Reich made outstanding contributions to the technique and theory of psychoanalysis."[56]

In any event, my analysis with Stern did result in less intellectualizing, more acting out, and a greater stirring of anxiety. The result was a separation from my wife and family, which was followed by a divorce and a move to the West several years later. At the time, divorce among psychoanalysts, or psychiatrists, was met with a degree of opprobium, for those in the field led, in a sense, a somewhat cloistered professional life; their social relations were chiefly with each other.

The gulf that divided the analytic fraternity from other specialists rested on a mystique that was partly verbal, partly ideological. Even our cousins, the neuropsychiatrists, appeared to be edgy when they were in earshot of conversations between analysts, using such terms as penis envy, clitoral orgasm, masturbation equivalent, or infantile erotism. Those of us who were candidates in psychoanalysis reveled in the freedom to fantasize, to interpret, and to rise above our former classmates into a realm where intuition rather than biophysical reality ruled.

Immersed in psychoanalytic detail, we paid little attention to studies like that of Abraham Myerson in 1939 in which he sent out 428 questionnaires to neurologists, psychiatrists, and psychologists (307 of whom answered) requesting that they state whether they (a) accepted psychoanalysis, (b) were favorably inclined toward it with some skepticism, (c) rejected psychoanalytic tenets, or (d) rejected with the view that psychoanalysis hindered progress in mental diseases.[57] Myerson found the opinions to be almost equally divided, 47 percent negative and 49 percent positive; his general conclusion was that "psychoanalysis had failed to prove its worth" as a therapeutic measure.

Of course such animadversions never reached our ears, for the training at the institute was quite thorough and absorbed our full vigilance. The seminars, for example, began with a careful reading of the five volumes of Freud's *Collected Works,* a veritable Pentateuch of psychoanalysis in its early development. Studies by Abraham, Jones, Ferenczi, Glover, and others, were reviewed with the aid of the seminar leaders who were outstanding analysts in New York—Sandor Lorand, Bertram Lewin, Abram Kardiner, Sandor Rado, George Daniels, and Phyllis Greenacre. These individuals gave of their time and energy to instruct us in the myriad connections between the unconscious and its representation in symptoms. Study groups and seminars were held in the institute on West Eighty-sixth Street. The building lay in the midst of a row of commodious dwellings of the 1905 era that had been converted by extending the spacious parlor into a small auditorium and the upper floor chambers room into conference rooms. Classes held in the evening often lasted until 11 P.M., as the instructors offered bits of material from their cases for the interpretation and free association of the students. After classes we would mull over the complexities of the analytic procedure and our reactions to the seminar leaders in a coffee shop on Broadway.

The continuous case seminars in which the changes in the case under discussion were followed week by week, allowing free play for the student's associations and comments augmented by the leader's reactions were extremely helpful. Thus, the whole gamut of analytic experience—analysis of dreams, movements of the ego in response to unconscious drives, instinctual transformation, the pleasure principle, analysis of sadistic and masochistic elements, repetition compulsions, castration derivatives, reaction formations, countertransference of the analyst—was laid bare, worked over, and interpreted. It was intense and heady fare that equipped the student to proceed with an analysis of his own cases under the control of a supervising analyst on the faculty.

CHANGES IN THE PSYCHOANALYTIC SCENE

Not only the classes but even the monthly society meetings filled our ears with analytic material. Every conceivable problem received an airing at the meeting, including cultural anthropology. The speakers were inspiring: Sandor Rado, René Spitz, Bertram Lewin, Philip Lehrman, Geza Roheim, and Gregory Zilboorg discussed the papers before the assembly, bringing out nuances, viewpoints, and shades of opinion in a dazzling array. I recall one meeting at which Lewin presented his analysis of elation. In the following discussion Zilboorg lauded the rich clinical feast of

analytic interpretation Lewin's communication afforded, but satisfaction in the intellectual tour de force and loyalty to analytic
tradition was destined to fragment.

The initiating occasion was the invitation to Karen Horney
in 1939 to address the society. Her speech opened a schism in
the analytic ranks. A handsome gray-haired woman, speaking
calmly at first without affectation, she discussed her dissatisfaction
with Freud's understanding of feminine psychology, his libido
theory, and his lack of consideration for cultural and social
stresses on the growing individual. As the talk progressed she
became visably emotional. Her address virtually renounced the
entire Freudian metapsychology—the notion of penis envy, the
importance of evoking infantile memories, and so forth. The
attack represented a definite break in the Freudian ranks. Within
a year it led several like-minded analysts to secede from the society,
which resulted in a rupture of the New York analytic fraternity.

Horney's devaluation of many Freudian ideas, which was
amplified in her 1939 book *New Ways in Psychoanalysis*, led to
counterattacks.[58] In response to her attack, Otto Fenichel, presumably representing the American Psychoanalytic Association's
stance, wrote, "What Horney wants to do is to abolish the essence
of psychoanalysis . . . by her distrust of rigid technical terms
[that] have become Frankensteins . . . obstructing our view of
the emotions and defenses as they occur in neurotic patients."[59]
Her frontal criticism of the cardinal points in Freudian analysis
included the passive "mirror" attitude of the analyzer, anxiety
as the result of the unconscious stimuli impinging on the ego,
reconstruction of the patient's childhood memories, and the mascu-
line sexual emphasis in Freud's axiom "anatomy is destiny." In
place of these principles, she advanced a "constructive friendliness"
on the part of the therapist, a *basic anxiety* ("the intrinsic weakness and helplessness [of the child] toward a potentially hostile
and dangerous world"), attention to real social factors in the
patient's life, and a rejection of the male view of penis envy
in female psychology.[60] Little wonder that Fenichel wrote "her
wish to outgrow the limitations of instinct and genetic psychology
is completely opposite the significance and value of psychoanalysis." Alexander reacted similarly: "Horney tried to create the

effigy of a one-sided biologically oriented Freud. Then, in order to destroy this effigy, she became extremely one-sided in the opposite direction."[61]

The meeting at the New York Psychoanalytic Institute was historic in that it signaled the "ferment taking place in American psychoanalysis in the late thirties," as Judd Marmor put it in 1973.[62] Horney's attack on male chauvinism, a phrase not current at that time, had an undoubted effect on the traditional posture and behavior of analysts, softening some, hardening others. In 1941 it actually split analytic ranks with the organization of the Association for the Advancement of Psychoanalysis and Psychosomatic Medicine in New York in which Rado, Kardiner, Janet Rioch, George Daniels, and others were prominent members.

With the crumbling of traditional analytic solidarity, new approaches developed. The key criterion of analytic work "to make conscious the unconscious" was replaced by Alexander's "corrective emotional experience."[63] Over the years there had been much questioning of the actual therapeutic effect of psychoanalysis, and at this turning point, therapists began to examine the necessity of long-term treatment. Some analysts accepted a lengthy period of treatment, from five to ten years, as the mark of thoroughness. Oberndorf remarked on "the trend of discussion in psychoanalytic meetings . . . that long analyses are desirable and presumably the most effective."[64] In his usual gentle manner, he hinted that "possibly too great or too deep preoccupation with the unconscious [may] retard the synthesis between conscience and primitive drives." Franz Alexander, sensing the same impasse, was more direct.[65] Impressed with the need to dissolve the protracted dependence some patients developed, he recommended short-term treatment, the so-called brief analysis. Simultaneously some of the traditional passivity of the analyst was being reduced through Paul Federn's suggestion of a closer appreciation of the reality of the treatment situation by a "nourishment of the transference through sincerity and kindness," an idea originally advanced by Ferenczi.[66] These modifications and fragmentations in the original analytic associations (New York, Washington, Baltimore), resulting in independent groups—the Association for the Advancement of Psychoanalysis, the Society of Medical

Psychoanalysts, the Association for Psychoanalytic and Psychosomatic Medicine, later the American Academy of Psychoanalysis—barely concerned the majority of candidates.

Our task as candidates was to engage in the supervised analysis of our patient, complete our own analysis, read a paper before the society, and apply for membership. The process seemed straightforward but obstacles could and did arise. Under supervision, the candidate brought the material gathered from the five-days-a-week treatment of his patient to his supervisor for a weekly conference covering technique, patient and therapist reactions, understanding of unconscious derivatives, and so forth. The case I worked on was a young physician, a resident in pediatrics at Willard Parker Hospital, who was overwhelmed by depression and feelings of insecurity. For months I followed the material he presented, making interpretations in consonance with what I had learned. No changes appeared in my patient's behavior or complaints. My analyst suggested that my own mounting anxiety interfered with the therapeutic efforts. Actually, a rearrangement in my life pattern, a rupture of family ties accompanied by a strong desire to leave the tense situation in New York for the West, lay behind this anxiety. The supervised analysis limped along for a few more weeks when the educational committee advised me to engage another control analyst.

Clara Thompson, before she split with the New York group along with Karen Horney, was selected. Accordingly, in the weekly sessions, I presented a second case on which I was working. She listened amiably but made no interpretations or comments about my technique. A few more sessions droned along when the sessions came to a halt. Nothing of any consequence happened to bring the supervisory sessions to a close. Dr. Thompson was pleasant but not informative; one under analysis is never quite sure what is happening. Shortly thereafter the committee recommended another supervising analyst.

On this occasion the distinguished Heinz Hartmann, who had recently emigrated from Europe, was suggested. A tall, sober man, whom Roazen had called the "American prime minister of analysis," listened gravely, said little, and presently these sessions too ceased without reproof or explanation.[67] The Kafka-like atmosphere was somewhat unnerving. I reported the denouement to Stern who said something to the effect that one could not observe the bottom of a stream if the waters were muddied; perhaps "muddled" would have been more appropriate. In any case, I took this to mean that the analysis would have to await clarification of my personal situation.

But the wheel of history took a hand in this period of strain and confusion. Two days after my analytic relapse, December 7, 1941, the attack on Pearl Harbor astounded the nation. I left New York City the following day. Pearl Harbor Day became a turning point in American history. It also served as a turning point in American psychiatry.

NOTES

1. National Committee on Mental Hygiene, "Surrey," *Mental Hygiene* 19, no. 2 (April 1935): 332.

2. Harold Palmer and Frank J. Braceland, "Six Years Experience with Narcosis Therapy," *American Journal of Psychiatry* 94 (July 1937): 37.

3. Kenneth Appel, C. B. Farr, and F. J. Braceland, "The Aschner Treatment of Schizophrenia: A Therapeutic Note," *American Journal of Psychiatry* 92 (July 1935): 201-6.

4. Manfred Sakel, "A New Treatment of Schizophrenia," *American Journal of Psychiatry* 93 (January 1937): 829.

5. Manfred Sakel, "Report of 89th Meeting of the Swiss Psychiatric Association, 1937" *American Journal of Psychiatry* 94 (May 1938): Supplement 24-40.

6. Joseph Wortis, *Fragments of an Analysis with Freud* (New York: Simon & Schuster, 1954), p. 110.

7. Bernard Glueck, Personal communication, circa 1937.

8. Joseph Wortis, et al., "Further Experience at Bellevue Hospital with Insulin Treatment in Schizophrenia," *American Journal of Psychiatry* 94 (July 1937): 152.

9. Sakel, "Report of the 89th Meeting."

10. Committee on Public Education, "Insulin Shock Treatment for Schizophrenia," *American Journal of Psychiatry* 93 (January 1937): 985-86.

11. See L. J. Von Meduna, "Pharmaco-dynamic Treatment of Psychoneurosis," *Diseases of the Nervous System* 8 (1947): 37-40;

Ugo Carletti, "Old And New Information About Electroshock," *American Journal of Psychiatry* 107 (August 1950):87.

12. L. B. Kalinowsky and H. Hippius, *Pharmaco-psychiatry* (New York: Grune & Stratton, 1969).

13. John Frosch and David Impastato, "Effects of Shock Treatment on the Ego," *Psychoanalytic Quarterly* 17 (1948): 226.

14. Kalinowsky & Hippius, *Pharmaco-psychiatry*, p. 32.

15. Otto Fenichel, *The Psychoanalytic Theory of Neurosis* (New York: W. W. Norton, 1945), p. 554.

16. Ira S. Wile, "Integration of the Child, The Goal of the Education Program," *Mental Hygiene* 20, no. 2 (April 1936): 249-61.

17. "Comment," *Mental Hygiene* 20, no. 3 (July 1936): 532.

18. Elizabeth J. Adamson, *So You're Going to a Psychiatrist* (New York: Thomas Crowell Co., 1936).

19. Harry Tiebout, "Address at New York University, Conference on Handicapped Children During the Depression," *Mental Hygiene* 18, no. 2 (April 1934): 323.

20. Abraham H. Maslow, *Toward a Psychology of Being,* 2d ed. (New York: Van Nostrand Co., 1968); Maslow, *The Farther Reaches of Human Nature* (New York: Viking Press, 1971).

21. Otto Rank, *Will Therapy and Truth and Reality,* trans. J. Taft (New York: Alfred A. Knopf, 1945).

22. Donald L. Burnham, "Orthodoxy and Eclecticism. Eclecticism in Psychoanalysis: The Washington-Baltimore Experience," in *American Psychoanalysis,* ed. J. Quen and C. T. Carlson (New York: Brunner Mazel, 1978), p. 87.

23. Alfred Korzybski, *Science and Sanity* (New York: International University Press, 1933).

24. Alfred Korzybski, "Neuro-semantic and Neuro-linguistic Mechanisms," *American Journal of Psychiatry* 92 (July 1936):28.

25. Markus Reiner, "Review of Science and Sanity," *Psychoanalytic Quarterly* 3 (1934): 641.

26. Harry S. Sullivan, "The Language of Schizophrenia," in *Language and Thought in Schizophrenia,* ed. J. Kasanin, (Berkeley: University of California Press, 1944), pp. 4-15.

27. Norman Cameron, "Experimental Analysis of Schizophrenic Thinking," in *Language and Thought in Schizophrenia,* pp. 50-63.

28. Kurt Goldstein, "Methodogical Approach to the Study of Schizophrenic Thought Disorder," in *Language and Thought in Schizophrenia,* pp. 17-39.

29. Jacob Kasanin and Eugenia Hanfmann, "An Experimental Study of

Concept Formation in Schizophrenia," *American Journal of Psychiatry* 95, no. 1 (July 1938): 35.

30. S. J. Beck, "Errors in Perception and Fantasy in Schizophrenics," in *Language and Thought in Schizophrenia,* p. 91.

31. John B. Watson, *Behavior, Introduction to Comparative Psychology,* (New York: Holt, Rinehart & Winston, 1967).

32. Alan E. Kazdin, *History of Behavior Modification*, (Baltimore: University Park Press, 1978), p. 309.

33. Joseph Wolpe, *The Conditioning Therapies* (New York: Holt, Rinehart & Winston, 1966).

34. Albert Moll, *A Lifetime of Mental Healing,* trans. (Dresden: Carl Reisser, 1936). Reviewed by Fritz Wittels, *Psychoanalytic Quarterly* 7 (1938): 267.

35. Josephine Jackson, *Guiding Your Life* (New York: Appelton-Century, 1937). Reviewed by Phyllis Greenacre, *Psychoanalytic Quarterly* 7 (1938): 286.

36. Franz Alexander, "Psychoanalysis Comes of Age," *Psychoanalytic Quarterly* 7 (1938): 299.

37. Adolf Meyer, "Subject Organization, Fourth Conference on Psychiatric Education (1936)," in *The Commonsense Psychiatry of Dr. Adolf Meyer,* ed. Alfred Lief (New York: McGraw-Hill, 1948), p. 618.

38. Abraham Myerson, "Theory and Principles of the 'Total Push' Method in the Treatment of Chronic Schizophrenia," *American Journal of Psychiatry* 95 (1939): 1197.

39. W. A. Bryan, "Re-education of Demented Patients," *American Journal of Psychiatry* 77 (1920): 99.

40. Samuel Atkin, "The New York Psychoanalytic Society and Institute: Its Founding and Development," in *American Psychoanalysis: Origins and Development,* ed. J. Quen and E. T. Carlson (New York: Brunner/Mazel, 1978), p. 73.

41 Personal communication.

42. A. A. Brill, "Abraham Lincoln as a Humorist" (Paper delivered at joint session of American Psychiatry Association and American Psychoanalytic Association, Toronto, Canada, June 1931).

43. Note on the Toronto meeting of the American Psychiatry Association, *Psychiatric Quarterly* 5 (1931): 609.

44. Clarence Oberndorf, *The History of Psychoanalysis in America* (New York: Grune & Stratton, 1953), p. 188.

45. Ibid.

46. Ibid., p. 30.

47. Abram Kardiner, "Frontiers of Psychology, Report on 1974

Meeting of American Academy of Psychoanalysts," *Roche Report,* 1 February 1974.

48. Melitta Schmeideberg "After the Analysis," *Psychoanalytic Quarterly* 7 (1938): 122.

49. New York Psychoanalytic Institute, "Regulations," *Psychoanalytic Quarterly* 7 (1938): 294.

50. Ibid., p. 295.

51. Eugen Kahn, *Psychopathic Personalities,* trans. H. Flanders Dunbar (New Haven: Yale University Press, 1931), pp. 62, 312.

52. Ernest G. Lion and Eugen Kahn, "Experimental Aspects of Huntington's Chorea," *American Journal of Psychiatry* 95 (November 1938): 717.

53. Adolph Stern, "Psychoanalytic Investigation of and Therapy in the Border Line Group of Neuroses," *Psychoanalytic Quarterly* 7 (1938): 246.

54. Wilhelm Reich, "On Character Analysis (1928)," trans. R. Fleiss, in *The Psychoanalytic Reader,* ed. Robert Fleiss, (New York: International University Press, 1948), 1:129-47.

55. Wilhelm Reich, *Orgonomic Diagnosis of Cancer Biopathy* (Orgonon, Me.: Orgone Institute Press, 1952).

56. Martin Grotjahn, "Review of Reich's *Die Bione,* 1938," *Psychoanalytic Quarterly* 7 (1938): 568.

57. Abraham Myerson, "The Attitude of Neurologists, Psychiatrists and Psychologists Towards Psychoanalysis," *American Journal of Psychiatry* 96 (1939): 623.

58. Karen Horney, *New Ways in Psychoanalysis* (New York: W. W. Norton Co., 1939).

59. Otto Fenichel, "Review of Horney's *New Ways in Pschoanalysis,*" *Psychoanalytic Quarterly* 9 (1940): 114.

60. Horney, *New Ways in Psychoanalysis,* p. 77 et seq.

61. Franz Alexander and S. T. Selesnick, *The History of Psychiatry* (New York: Harper & Row, 1966), p. 366.

62. Judd Marmor, Newsletter, WAWI, 1973, quoted in "Organizational Schisms in American Psychoanalysis," in *American Psychoanalysis,* p. 147.

63. Judd Marmor, *The Contributions of Franz Alexander to Modern Psychotherapy* (Nutley, N.J.: LaRoche Co., 1972).

64. Clarence Oberndorf, "Factors in Psychoanalytic Therapy," *American Journal of Psychiatry* 98 (March 1942): 750.

65. Franz Alexander, *Psychoanalytic Therapy, Principles and Applications* (New York: Ronald Press, 1946).

66. Paul Federn, "Psychoanalysis of Psychoses," *Psychiatric Quarterly* 17 (1943): 3, 245, 470.

67. Paul Roazen, *Freud and his Followers* (New York: Alfred A. Knopf, 1975), p. 520.

7

A TURNING POINT

As the 1930s came to an end, it is safe to say that the new generation of psychiatrists had incorporated psychoanalytic ideation in their thinking. Psychiatrists trained in the larger centers, such as New York, Washington-Baltimore, Boston, and Chicago, regarded those defense mechanisms arising from the unconscious as indisputable elements in psychopathology. The techniques used in therapy were aimed at uncovering mechanisms of repression, projection, introjection, displacement, and so forth. More significantly, the literate public had become convinced of the need for a "depth" analysis to cure neurosis, character distortions, and even marital, sexual, and economic maladjustments in life. Psychoanalysis was expected to illuminate every aspect of human endeavor, including international affairs and politics. It was generally agreed, in spite of the cavil of some in the field, that Freud's metapsychology rested on the firm basis of his meticulous observations of patients under treatment. But the acceptance of unconscious dynamics did not answer the question of whether or not patients were actually cured by the Freudian technique. Obviously, professional therapists needed a theoretical structure to guide them in their work. Theorizing is a necessity for the therapist; an interesting but secondary enterprise for the patient.

PSYCHOANALYSIS CRITICIZED

The early opposition to psychoanalysis, either on the grounds of morality (the sexual accent was offensive to some) or science (logic), became less urgent in the face of the nagging question of curative efficiency. Furthermore, as analysis spread in popularity, questions arose concerning its cost in time and money and its applicability to a legion of neurotic sufferers throughout the country. Coincidentally, neuropsychiatrists and psychosomatically oriented physicians who had referred cases to analysts became disenchanted with anecdotal accounts of cures. They wished for an answer to the more pointed question of its therapeutic value. Abraham Myerson's conclusion that analysis was ineffective as a healing agent was echoed by a report of two competent internists in New York, Leo Kessel and Harold Hyman who in 1933 had referred a group of thirty-three patients to various analysts.[1] Their cases included homosexual, schizophrenic, depressed, neurotic, and psychosomatic patients. They found that after an appropriate treatment time, seventeen of the thirty-three were "distinctly benefitted . . . and 16 . . .dismal failures." Three years later, Hyman added ten more cases with similar findings; his experiences prompted him to write disapprovingly in a 1936 *Journal of the American Medical Association* that "the literature of psychoanalysis, opulent in its imagery and broad vistas of potentialities offers little tangible clinical information."[2]

Hyman's criticism neglected to take into account the difficult problems of deciding on the extent of a "cure," the variations in diagnoses and in symptoms, the length of time after analytic treatment, the personalities of the several analysts, and other intricate problems in defining the social, marital, economic, or psychosexual cure or improvement after analytic treatment. This task, with all its caveats, was attempted in 1941 by Robert Knight of the Menninger Clinic.[3] His study of 952 cases derived from reports of the Berlin Institute (1920-1930), the London Clinic (1926-1936), the Chicago Institute (1932-1937), the Menninger Clinic (1932-1941), and Hyman and Kessler's New York Group was a heroic effort, considering the different diagnoses and criteria of cure employed. Of the composite reports on 952 patients, Knight concluded that psychoanalysis was "effective" for the psychoneuroses, sexual disorders, and organ neuroses and showed "some promise" for the addictions and psychoses.

Meanwhile, the treatment for psychotic persons, schizophrenics and depressives, and later severely obsessive and compulsive patients, continued to involve shock methods—Metrazol and insulin coma—to a growing chorus of approval. Much later, in 1966, Hans Hoff of the University of Vienna, who had watched Sakel develop his insulin shock method, remarked at an international conference of the Manfred Sakel Foundation, "Psychiatry often oscillates with passing fashions like reeds in the wind," but Sakel's method "changed the course of psychiatry."[4] Reports of treatment with Metrazol, and then a combination of Metrazol and insulin, filled the *Journal of the American Psychiatric Association*. The popularity of shock methods usually arose from reports of small groups of patients. On a larger canvas, J. F. Bateman and Nicholas Michael studied a large group by collating all the shock treatments used in the Ohio state hospital system for the years 1937 to 1938. They found of 416 patients treated with insulin shock, 130 recovered and 29 showed improvement.[5] Of 579 patients treated with Metrazol, 88 recovered and 199 improved; of a control group of 325 untreated cases, 49 recovered and 79 improved. They concluded that insulin treatment is "justified . . . Metrazol is disappointing." On a still larger scale John Ross and his associates reported on 1,757 patients treated with insulin in the New York state hospital system for a similar period. They concluded that insulin shock therapy was the "best single therapeutic measure . . . since 75% of treated patients . . . retained benefit status after two years."[6]

The popularity of Sakel's innovation during these years can be gauged by Kolb and Vogel's nationwide tabulation of 66,688 patients treated in state, federal, and private hospitals from 1935 to 1941 with insulin (23,651), Metrazol (38,839), and the newly introduced electroshock (7,769).[7] Within a few years electroshock surpassed Metrazol as the choice of treatment for depressions and other psychotic conditions. With improvements in technique—curare for eliminating traumatic hazards (that is, fractures and dislocations), preliminary administration of Amytal to reduce anxiety, subcoma insulin treatment for neurotic and toxic states, electroshock in the office—the use of electroshock grew enormously after World War II.[8] During the prewar years, however, electroshock as the primary method of reducing the length of hospitalization and of minimizing the anguish of depressed patients had not yet gained a favored position.

PREWAR EXPERIENCES

The increasingly ominous developments in Europe were not reflected immediately in the field of psychiatry, except that they resulted in a resettlement, chiefly in New York City, of prominent psychoanalysts from Germany and Austria. The early group of expatriates, Rado, Schilder, Wittels, Lorand, and Feigenbaum, who had heeded the rumble of the distant drum before 1933, were reinforced by those who came after 1933. A committee of the New York Psychoanalytic Institute embarked on a program to rescue analysts from Teutonic destructiveness that resulted in the subsequent settlement of such leaders as Hartmann, Bychowski, Kris, Spitz, Roheim, Loewenstein, and Bergler in New York. These importations enriched psychoanalysis, accentuated its influence on psychiatry, and gave form to the structure of psychoanalytic institutes in the major centers.

The impact of events in Europe exerted little influence on psychiatric research and practice in this country during the late 1930s. But there were deep-seated psychological reactions among the public; there was a growing irritation and anger at the strident voice of Hitler and his aides and the pomposity of Mussolini. As stories of repression and disenfrachisement filtered through in the tales of emigrés, the conclusion that Hitler was paranoid, possibly psychotic, met with general agreement. The Anschlüss with Austria and the sudden turn against the Soviet Union in 1939 only confirmed the diagnosis. Psychiatric interest in Teutonic folk psychology increased. Richard Brickner, a Columbia neuropsychiatrist, discussed the background of what he called "German paranoid orientation . . . a significant part of German history."[9] He also showed how Hitlerian doctrine evolved from this preoccupation. "German supremacy," he noted, "is a longstanding progressive paranoid trend."

Curiously enough, the psychiatric fraternity in New York at least, published relatively little about the Nazi anti-Semitism that roiled a large part of American citizenry. Dorian Feigenbaum, himself an emigré, mentioned the subject briefly in a long paper, entitled "On Projection," which appeared in the *Psychoanalytic Quarterly* in 1936.[10] He described anti-Semitism as the "projection

of repressed (displaced) aggressivity . . . while on the other hand
the Jews' awareness of anti-Semitism . . . may . . . be based not so
much on actual reality as on a projection of his own unconscious
hostility towards non-Jews." Otto Fenichel addressed himself
to the "scapegoat" theory of anti-Semitism, citing it as a projection by "the oppressed non-Jewish population in Germany,"
who then use the Jew as a "target for their own resentment
against their oppressors."[11]

As Hitler's *Judenfrei* plan (to free the world of Jews) became
a stark reality, the psychoanalytic fraternity sought to clean its
house by accusing Jung of supporting the Nazi cause. His studies
of cultural symbolism and archetypes, some of which have racial
characteristics, were taken as proof of his Hitlerian leanings.
In his work *The Integration of Personality,* published in English
on 1939, Jung stated, "Great liberating deeds of world history
have come from leading personalities and never from the inert
mass . . . [who] need a demogogue if it is to move at all."[12]
To this and other remarks about the collective unconscious,
reviewer Ralph Kaufman, who reviewed the book for the *Psychoanalytic Quarterly*, wrote, "The final chapter . . . [contains] the
choicest anti-democratic thinking to be found outside the Ministry
of Propaganda."[13] The English psychoanalyst Edward Glover,
pointing to the unbridgeable chasm between Freudian and Jungian
analysis, quoted Jung in support of the Nazi leader: "Hitler's
first idea is to make his people powerful because the spirit of
the Aryan German deserves to be supported by might, muscle and
steel."[14] Whatever the truth of Jung's sympathies with National
Socialism before the war, his name remained under a cloud during
this period. The schism between Freud and Jung was, of course,
old history. In one of his works, Jung remarked of earlier days,
"Though recent experience I was deeply impressed by the almost
unbridgeable gap between Freud's mental outlook and background
and my own."[15] The recrudescence of this feud, which was stimulated by Nazi depredations, is an indication of how aggressive
impulses in the individual are aroused by a hostile world.

Psychiatry and psychiatrists were not unmoved by the rumblings
of the Axis powers from 1938 on. Even before President Roosevelt's
immediate declaration of war on December 7, 1941, the "day that

shall live in infamy," there had been some preparation among psychiatrists in Washington, D.C., for the seemingly inevitable confrontation. In 1939 the council of the American Psychiatric Association appointed a Committee on Military Mobilization under Harry A. Steckel to discover what psychiatric personnel would be available in case of need. But, as Albert Deutsch, the historian of American mental hygiene, remarked, "Leadership . . . [was] at first marked by hesitation and uncertainty of purpose."[16] Captain Dallas Sutton of the U.S. Navy Medical Corps was more direct. As he reported of his peace-time experience, "The most important mission of the peace-time combat organization . . . is that of preparation for war."[17] A southern psychiatric association committee emphasized the need to combat "a strategy of insecurity and fear," a task of morale building that fell on the shoulders of psychiatrists.[18] Anticipating a large number of recruits, the National Research Council developed a plan for mental examinations of draftees, which the Selective Service adopted.

In September 1940, the National Defense Program asked for 600 civilian, part-time officer psychiatrists to help in military hospitals.[19] By January 1941, Clarence Dykstra, chief of the Selective Service, recognized the importance of psychiatrists in the military to "eliminate psychiatric risks."[20]

As preparedness for the conflict grew, Lieutenant Colonel Roy Halloran was appointed chief of the Neuro-Psychiatric Division of the Surgeon General's Office, to be followed, on his death, by Colonel William Menninger. Plans for a wide range of psychiatric services, along the lines developed by Edward Strecker in World War I, were put into action. The induction stations, training areas, staging areas, and finally combat sectors all demanded psychiatric expertise. Judging by the flood of papers in the *American Journal of Psychiatry,* the problems confronting psychiatric officers fell into every area of human behavior. To cite only one example, Wilfred Bloomberg and Robert Hyde, concerned with neurotic and psychopathic personalities who presented "greater than average risk of breaking down under the strain of army service," reported their experiences at the Boston induction station in July 1942.[21] By the end of 1942 the journal had published many articles, ranging from "Social Data in Psychiatric Casualities" to the full array of military problems that faced the neurologist and psychiatrist.[22] These covered the usual neuroses and psychoses faced in civil practice, as well as such special situations as chronic exhaustion in test pilots, combat fatigue, hysterical episodes, personality disorders among soldiers, etc.

It became evident that the supply of specialists was inadequate to meet military needs; crash courses in military neuropsychiatry (six weeks of intensive lectures and seminars) were instituted for the so-called sixty day wonders, many of whom remained in the psychiatric field after the war.[23] (Edward Strecker had arranged a similar rapid-training plan for a limited number of doctors during World War I.) As the war ground on, military needs changed. Norman Brill best described the development: Up to 1943 induction and training constituted the chief area for psychiatric expertise; from then to the end of the conflict, hospitalization and discharge problems, including Veteran's Administration cases, engaged psychiatrists.[24] The annual meeting of the American Psychiatric Association in spring of 1943 featured a symposium of prominent psychiatrists in the army, navy, air force, Merchant Marines, and Public Health Service.[25] Colonel Roy Halloran, Malcolm Farrell, Franklin Ebaugh, Leon J. Saul, Howard Rome, Bernard Cruvant, Daniel Blain, Henry Brosin, and many more discussed the entire gamut of nervous disorders in the serviceman. These problems tested the ingenuity and dedication of American psychiatry.

Prewar Civil Psychiatry

The practice of civilian psychiatry changed little during the early period of the war. There was perhaps less emphasis on psychoanalysis. Karl Menninger, as president of the American Psychoanalytic Association at its annual meeting in May 1942, counseled its members: "The Army, the Navy, and the Public Health Service, recognize psychiatry; they do not recognize psycho-analysis. . . . It behooves us to pay prime attention to our patients and not attempt to get a foothold in political or governmental activities."[26] The primary emphasis in civilian practice remained the biochemistry of the brain, in part as the consequence of the puzzling success of shock therapies.[27] Other problems attracted attention as well: the neuropathology of the senile states; the use of vitamins in alcoholic toxic conditions; epilepsy, and the newly developed drug, Dilantin; lobotomy; Korzybski's *General Semantics*; the hereditary-constitutional basis of mental disease. Of the numerous clinical problems under study, that of traumatic neurosis, developed by Kardiner in his *Bio-Analysis of the Epileptic Reaction,* and amplified among veterans of World War I, became particularly important for World War II psychiatrists.[28]

Another field of clinical psychiatry, one dealing with the two problems of the psychopathic character and criminally insane engaged the efforts of a slowly growing band of men. Alienists called to determine the insanity of those accused of capital offenses were increasingly the butt of citizens' complaints about the "battle of experts" in courts. In New York, as elsewhere, the lunacy commissions did not routinely include trained psychiatrists. During the late 1930s, the Blanshard Commission, which was organized to investigate the "obvious waste of money . . . in appointing lunacy commissions" for examination of offenders pleading insanity, branded them as "'gravy' for certain political pleading and their friends."[29] A bill signed by Governor Lehman, after a vote by a previous governor, abolished the existing lunacy commissions in New York State in 1939 and called for one member of each new commission to be a qualified psychiatrist, in place of the older system that used a physician, a lawyer, and a layman. During the early stages of the war, a few individual investigators continued their work with criminals, which was overshadowed by the growing problems of psychopaths in the military service.[30]

WARTIME PSYCHIATRY

My entry into military psychiatry occurred in an improbable place, Reno, Nevada. I had left my native New York for personal reasons the day after Pearl Harbor. The Overland Limited, which passed through Chicago and continued West, was filled with soldiers and sailors returning to their units. The atmosphere reflected their excitement as radio broadcasts told and retold of the feverish preparations in Washington. But the war excitement was absent when I detrained in Reno, a block from the rather modest gambling strip of Harold's Club fame. Here the imprint of the West was unmistakable. The measured pace of the small city—a few cowboys and tourist-divorcees, an occasional Indian ambling along Virginia Street in an unhurried, aimless manner—seemed to mirror the limits imposed by the Sierra-Nevada range surrounding the city. Something of the eternality of the mountains, drowsing contentedly under a cleansed sky, determined the atmosphere. Although despair and distraught emotions lay behind this apparent aimlessness, one had the sense of witnessing humans bravely facing an unadorned reality. Divorce attorneys were said to bring their anguished clients to Pyramid Lake to note how puny their troubles were compared to the vistas of distant mountains and the ungiving desert. On the surface it appeared to be a unique place for a psychiatrist.

Within a few weeks, I applied for a medical license, appeared before the state's medical examiners, and became the first psychiatrist in Nevada. Remarried, I embarked on practice, but psychiatry in such a hard-bitten area could be described as evanescent. Across the hall from my sparsely furnished office, a neurosurgeon, Charles Tranter, eked out a living by injecting depressed divorcees with sodium cacodylate to buoy up their frazzled nerves during the six-week waiting period. Although Tranter had had thorough training in Boston with Harry Solomon at the Boston Psychopathic and had spent some time in Harvey Cushing's clinic in neurosurgery, his specialism failed to impress the citizenry of Nevada at that time.

For a few weeks, I was semiofficially attached to the Washoe County General Hospital, whose psychiatric service was limited to two cells in the basement, chiefly for alcoholic delirium cases who "slept it off." Soon Tranter introduced me to a traveling Army team that performed induction examinations in remote parts of the state. Induction duty on a civilian status was a welcome respite from the unhurried ambience that was beginning to pall. With a colonel in charge, our small caravan visited desert towns, examined loose-limbed cowboys and taciturn Indians, and found little except alcoholism that could unfit them for service. Soon, the colonel invited me to San Francisco to the U.S. Army induction station for similar duties. During the next six months, working with Maier Tuchler, a neuropsychiatrist trained at Tulane University and Bellevue Hospital, I encountered thousands of youths and men, a modest number of whom were neurotic, defective, psychopathic, or psychotic. The number of selectees and recruits easily passed the limits set down by the special committee, which was headed by Winfred Overholser who recommended to the surgeon general in 1943 that "psychiatric examinations . . . be limited to fifty a day."[31] While our instructions to let no inadequate person slip by were dictated by the need for competent, trainable servicemen, they were also dictated by the real need to prevent the "tragic financial consequences of inadequate psychiatric examinations" and to teach local selection boards to realize the "significance of mental and personality factors."[32] Four hundred to five hundred individuals, hailing from the Far West, the desert, and the California valleys, passed through our unit per day. The material on which we placed our neurologic and psychiatric imprimatur varied: Frightened city youth, bewildered Chinese restaurant workers, mechanics, students, Bohemians, conscientious objectors, sophisticated San Franciscans, malingerers, and ranch workers from the "cow counties," passed in a steady stream to be diagnosed by a glance, perhaps a knee-jerk tap and a few questions. The few questionable cases were set aside for more careful examination at the end of the day. In spite of Deutsch's comment that the "two-minute average psychiatric interview at induction stations . . . proved little more than a farce," we felt we did a creditable job using experience rather than, as Deutsch claimed, "large sprinklings of hunches and fortune-telling."[33]

At the end of 1942, my commission in the naval reserve came through. I was assigned to the U.S. Naval Training Station in Farragut, Idaho, which was located on the plateau surrounding the enchanting Lake Pond Oreille. Our unit, commanded by Leon J. Saul, included Douglas Orr, a psychoanalyst from Seattle, Frances Gramlich, a psychologist-philosopher from Dartmouth College, a clinical psychiatrist from Texas, and a psychiatric social worker from Minneapolis. All of us were competent and eager to help the war effort. Trainloads of recruits from the Middle West and the West poured into the reception building to be inspected, auscultated, palpated, stethoscoped, tested for muscular defects, for genitourinary disorders, and finally dumped into small rooms where each psychiatrist sat unceremoniously, cataloguing them as fit or unfit for naval service. This done, the men, nude and carrying their possessions in a small canvas bag, slid down a chute, were dressed in Navy uniforms and emerged as men-of-war in a landlocked sea. Beside the assembly-line examinations, a few beds were detailed for panicky, anxious, enuretic recruits whose separation anxiety and depression were expressed in psychosomatic conditions. For four months, until a wheel turned in Washington, D. C., and orders came for me to travel to Pier 92, North River, New York City, our comradely group of psychiatrists and associates spent intense days and agreeable nights in this isolated mountain precinct.

The long pier, *sans* berthed ocean liners and empty of the usual cases, barrels, boxes of shipping material, and longshoremen, served temporarily as a receiving "ship" for the increasing number of antisocial problems that vexed military officers in the New York area. Servicemen on ships and staging areas within a one-hundred-mile radius of the city, made Broadway and Forty-second Street a haven for escape from overseas duty. Furloughs stretched to desertions, leaves to AWOL's, and the blandishments of New York's fleshpots and bars led to assaults, barroom brawls, and minor offenses. The military police who patrolled New York's "White Way" hauled men to the pier in such numbers that a larger barracks was needed. Hart's Island, a penitentiary wrested from the city that had once housed New York's drug addicts and petty thieves, filled the need. The navy appropriated the grounds bordering on Potter's field, raised the flag, cleaned out old red-bricked housing dormitories, refitted the galleys, secured the administration building for the command post, and awaited the hordes of men gathered in the shore patrol's nightly net.

Because desertions and AWOL's threatened to be a major problem, the judge advocate general and other naval authorities in Washington combed their personnel list for those experienced in criminology. My orders to Pier 92 to evaluate, and possibly rehabilitate or diagnose psychopaths unfit for duty, flowed from the directive to return "as many men to as many guns as possible"— the offical instructions of the Bureau of Medicine, Department of the U. S. Navy. My introduction to this diagnostic-morale-lifting duty was hardly fraternal. Captain Pashley, the crusty, old-line, commanding officer, surveyed me critically when I reported for duty. His instructions were brief, his commentary pointed. As I stood before the captain backed by a few staff officers standing behind him on the enormous empty pier, he said gruffly, "Surgeon, we don't want you [that is, psychiatrists] here but Washington sent you. I know how to handle men with shit in their veins." A few sympathetic words from the executive officer, a wink in the direction of the departing captain, and I found myself, hat in hand, standing alone on the huge pier.

Wartime Therapy

On Hart's Island, the reception of the commanding officer was noncommital. The line officers warily watched me as I set out to fulfill the mission of rehabilitation. The commander of the base, acknowledging that he knew nothing of psychiatry and cared less, assigned me a yeoman and a desk in a cubby hole. Fortunately within a few weeks, the executive officer decided psychiatrists were neither in league with Satan nor bound in brotherhood with Svengali. A larger space was given in the old visitors building of the penitentiary, and more staff was added, including a psychiatrist, two psychologists, a penal expert (a former probation officer), social workers, and a therapeutically minded Catholic chaplain with whom we worked closely. Our material consisted of frightened youths desperately trying to avoid the cold North Atlantic Murmansk run, where American merchant and naval vessels had been sunk by German U-boats; a few psychopaths inducted into the service; a body of authority-hating men who could not tolerate military discipline; and a large number of young men whose delight in a uniform soon evaporated in contact with the "sea gulls" of midtown New York. The use of marihuana, followed by apathy or criminal behavior, loomed as a major problem among naval personnel, as the young Americans who returned from ports in the Far East, Morocco, Algiers, or other African sea ports had been introduced to hashish, heroin, and other narcotic delights. The more the shore patrols hauled the men in, the more men were found hiding out. The naval command was observably concerned. One troublesome problem involved alliances with young women whose maternal instincts joined the servicemen's separation anxiety to mute the latter's desire to continue dangerous war duties.

Aside from examinations of rebellious prisoners, our main mission focused on rehabilitation with accent on implanting enthusiasm among the young prisoners for a war to vanquish Nazi and facist evil from the world. Aided by the line officers, we started with simple techniques: drilling men on the parade grounds bordering on Potter's field, the graveyard for New York's forgotten dead, which shared Hart's Island with the city reformatory. Nicknamed the "grinder," the miscreants were paraded endlessly on the field, often trampling underfoot an extruded skull or thigh bone from the mass graves. Soon a recreation department, made up of teachers, was added to help the sparsely educated men learn movie projection, develop a musical band, and so forth. With these aides we set to work to supply the necessary patriotism to our charges.

Triweekly meetings of the prisoners in a mess hall were arranged. Ship instructional films and navy films of Guadalcanal were shown, and the staff attempted to establish an atmosphere of camaraderie through discussions, simply told, of the meaning of separation anxiety and the emotional problems expected in military service. We interspersed our homey discussions, conceived of as a type of group therapy, with brief addresses by old "salts," veterans of South Seas encounters with Japanese aircraft and warships. One bosun's mate recalled how he lay on the beach covered with sand to escape strafing by Japanese planes that roared in from their carriers. The accounts were theatrical, sometimes lurid, and acted as an approach that we hoped would neutralize any fear of being "analyzed." This corridor opened, we encouraged the captive audience to voice their complaints of the staff, the food, and the conditions at the barracks—itself a shocking maneuver in the U. S. Navy. The response from the prisoners was silence. It became clear that we were not reaching the young offenders and equally clear that the problem lay in their hard-core opposition to authority. The loss to the service through their recalcitrancy was staggering. A statistical survey of 1,000 admissions to the installation demonstrated that ninety man-years of service were lost to the nation.[34] Of these offenders, 53 percent were repeaters, a finding that confirmed our frequent diagnosis of psychopathy.[35]

But diagnoses can be overdrawn; there were larger factors to be considered in the task of salvaging men for naval service in wartime. The war in the Pacific was costly for the navy, but the Atlantic area also inspired fear. The U-boat menace, in the words of Samuel Morison "knocked down ships like tenpins."[36] In two months, between May and June 1942, 182 ships were torpedoed by German submarines in the Atlantic, interrupting the passage of armies and supplies to Europe. Merchant ships sank in the North Atlantic when the temperature of the waters hovered around 30°F.[37] Desertions from merchant ships increased sharply. The cold waters on the Murmansk run brought psychic shivers to sailors assigned to that duty.

As disciplinary problems advanced to criminological ones— homicides, sexual perversions, assaults on officers, smuggling of narcotics from the Mediterranean ports—the Department of the Navy became even more concerned over this demoralization. In 1944 I was ordered to the U. S. Naval Prison at Portsmouth, New Hampshire. Whereas my associates and I at Hart's Island had functioned at captain's masts for minor infractions, now court martials imposed sentences for long stretches of hard labor. How much the grinding struggle of our country in midwar affected acting-out behavior remained a matter of speculation. Prisoners in the "Castle," as the old prison was called, represented a large group of ex-reformatory and penitentiary inmates who had slipped by the induction officers. Commanded by a Marine Corps colonel and a staff of Marine Corps veterans from Guadalcanal, discipline was harsh, and labor on the rock pile no empty threat. Indeed, the explosive reactions of the inmates often matched the mission of the prison.

The psychiatric staff, including Terry Rodgers, an analytically trained psychiatrist, and Fabian Rouke, a clinical psychologist from Manhattan College, examined the disturbed inmates, testified at court martials in Boston, and attended discharge conferences with officers of the line, where the problem concentrated on meting out dishonorable or bad conduct discharges to inmates returning to civilian life. In addition to these staff members, social and probation workers and chaplains were assigned to this duty. Again, I attempted a simple form of group therapy but aimed at the Marine Corps officers and men who formed the prison guard. This time we introduced the staff to the Rorschach test and discussed emotional dynamics in relation to antagonism to authority.[38] We spoke of aggression as a cover for dependence, of denial by the prisoners of their unperceived paternal identification to such a point that the term "emotional problem" supplanted harsher, and more salty characterizations, the hallmark of the Marine Corps. In the study of AWOL's at Hart's Island, Bernard Locke, Anthony Apuzzo, and I had found dependence needs of the servicemen, combined with resentment of authority to be major conflicts within the sailor who went AWOL. Applying this principle to the naval prisoners, our staff tried to supply a dynamic explanation to the military staff for the misfits and "yellow-bellied bastards" in the prison population.

Our commandant, Colonel Rossell, a man up from the ranks, understood our therapeutic aims. With his support, I attempted a modified analytic approach on one vicious nineteen-year-old prisoner who was insolent to the officers, destructive to the few furnishings in his cell, and defiant of all rules. Sentenced to the naval prison for theft and desertion, R. B. had been repeatedly diagnosed as a psychopathic personality. His background was rife with juvenile antisociality, his father an alcoholic whom he once met in the House of Corrections in his native city. Continued wildly destructive behavior in prison resulted in his orders for solitary confinement. Because the colonel permitted me to control punishment while he was under therapy, I ordered all punishment withheld and simultaneously ordered him to come for treatment daily. Placed on a cot in a room with barred windows, he grudgingly complied with the analytic rule. For the first month or two he was suffused with fantasies of crushing, smashing, or mangling the guards physically. Rage at the older staff took the form of their humiliation: "The gold braid have lived their lives. . . all they do is sit back and smoke cigars and control people," he said sneeringly. Contrary to prison regulations and the punitive instincts of the Marine guards, flurries of destruction in his cell after sessions with me were handled by again withholding punishment. One day he arrived with a "shiv," a long, sharpened piece of steel hidden in his sleeve. Threatening me, he said, "We are both getting out of here . . . in a box." Somehow I was able to calm his belligerence; suddenly his anger dissolved in tears. Again, punishment for the threatened assault on an officer, a serious offense, was withheld. In the weeks that followed, R. B.'s aggression decreased; his defended against dependency appeared in dreams and associations. One dream, which I reported in detail in the *Psychoanalytic Quarterly*, pictured his struggle with masochism: "A werewolf is wrestling with me. Then I am given a needle, and I'm supposed to stick it in my arm to poison me."[39] On the tier he began to defend against his fellow prisoners' taunts that he was a "fairy . . . in love with the psycho doc." With continued therapy, R. B. became interested in magazine articles portraying psychiatrists in the movies. Destructiveness dwindled; the inmate was more tractable until therapy was discontinued with my return to civilian status.

The problems in the navy during this time approximated those in other theatres of operation. The journals published articles covering the psychiatric experiences of men in the various campaigns. From induction station to combat zones, from the morale of the troops on occupation duty, to soldiers invalidated by shells, the whole gamut of mental and emotional disorders in war lay stretched out before American psychiatrists. As Carl Jonas well put it, psychiatrists reported on their "buffeting and unsettling experiences" in a flood of papers and books.[40] Roy Grinker and John Spiegel wrote of their heroic work with combat fliers in the Tunisian campaign using narcosynthesis to induce a relief from terror and reactions under German fire;[41] Manfred Guttmacher and Frank Stewart discussed the deserter problem in the army and concluded that "most men who go AWOL are psychiatrically abnormal."[42] Lewis Loeser wrote on sexual psychopaths, chiefly homosexuals, in military service;[43] George C. Burns described the neurotic reactions encountered on a lonely Aleutian outpost where, "some men not in combat developed combat fatigue" like their embattled brethren.[44] Bernard Diamond and Alice Ross related their experiences with 150 recently blinded soldiers;[45] David Rothschild reviewed 1,000 cases in a rear installation caring for veterans of South Pacific engagements.[46] Joseph Knapp and Frederick Weitzen described their rehabilitative efforts—push therapy—in a rehabilitation center at Fort Knox.[47]

Abstracting a few reports from far-flung lines conveys only a fraction of the war efforts of American psychiatrists. Guttmacher, in a review of the consultation services in the army, indicated the extent of these services and the reaction of senior officers: "older army officers . . . expressed great skepticism . . . [feeling that] consideration of the individual soldier was basically wrong."[48] The foundation of mental hygiene and psychiatry in their emphasis on the individual as a living, adjusting human being ran contrary to men bred in the tradition of controlling large bodies of robots. It "put ideas in their heads . . . which might lead to epidemics of malingery," they complained. The high command in the field of battle did report "numerous cases of SIW [self-inflicted wounds]" according to one of General Eisenhower's aides.[49] In a report of a division general to headquarters in 1944, "1,100 SIW cases" occurred in one drive on the western front. Still, the face-slapping incident of a hospitalized soldier by General Patton aroused Eisenhower to reprimand Patton for "routing several patients by the scruff of the neck . . . [and his use] of salty, expressive and colorful speech."[50]

Combating the groundswell of opposition to the individual handling of men by those who thought in terms of "available units" for military action concerned many psychiatrists on military duty. "Malingery," Guttmacher noted, "was not an important aspect" of psychiatric casualties in the army. What we all witnessed in varying degrees was the impact of an enterprise devoted to destruction of men and property on servicemen of many cultural backgrounds and personality formations. I recall a session one night at the prison when a member of the ship's company bitterly condemned the war because of the waste of steel to the world in the sinking of American ships in the Pacific—a curious displacement of anger and frustration on the part of a sailor.

The reactions of psychiatrists themselves to the war effort varied widely. Some awakened to the presence of a serious neurotic potential in our population as they witnessed the breaking point in ostensibly stable individuals under wartime stresses. Others found their training in peacetime psychiatry far from adequate in emergency situations. Thus, Jonas declared in his 1945 paper, entitled "Psychiatry Has Growing Pains," "We have learned that it is hard to renounce old training and beliefs though some of them were barren."[51] Although a good number of military doctors slipped back into clinical harness and regarded war experiences as unique, not to be duplicated in civilian life, younger medical officers embraced the specialty of psychiatry with enthusiasm. William Menninger, by 1945 a brigadier general in the surgeon general's office, breathed new life into psychiatry as the result of his war experiences. In 1946 he organized the Group for the Advancement of Psychiatry, whose aim was to "collect and appraise significant data in the field of psychiatry . . . for the promotion of mental health and good human relations." Known as the "young Turks," leaders in certain fields banded in small working committees to engage such problems as social issues, therapy, psychiatry in industry, preventive psychiatry, international relations, sexual psychopathy, and forensic psychiatry. I was a member of the latter group for a few years. White papers covering the several fields of interest were published; experts in kindred areas, anthropologists, sociologist, lawyers, educators, economists, biologists, were freely called on for advice. The group's acronym, GAP, was hailed as a leading edge of psychiatric progress.

Then came Hiroshima, V-J Day, and V-E Day.

Judging by Paul Hoch's review "Psychiatric Progress," published in the *American Journal of Psychiatry* in 1945, with the war's end, psychiatry in the civilian sector had advanced on all fronts.[52] He detailed categories of progress: research activities; physiological treatment of psychoses; alcohol; geriatrics; neurosyphilis; child psychiatry; mental deficiency; heredity and eugenics; epilepsy; biochemistry, endocrinology and neuropathology; family care; outpatient clinics; psychiatric social work; administrative, forensic, and military psychology; psychiatric education; and psychometrics. New medications, new methods, new techniques crowded the psychiatric scene.

L'ENVOI

How will history judge the decades outlined here? Just as the nineteenth century produced understanding of mental diseases through the classification of the insanities, so the twentieth century advanced to an analysis of the mental life behind mental illness. Was this period a way station or a terminus to man's quest for a final answer to mental disorders? In truth, both these enterprises brought enlightenment; they also brought a kind of quiet despair that mental and nervous diseases were fixed attributes of human life. But the period between the wars evoked different attitudes. The vigorous winds of mental health and an interpretive psychiatry swept away some of this passivity, this nihilism in the face of mental disorder. In so doing, it formed an admixture that vitalized psychiatry.

The swing into a psychological psychiatry was undoubtedly stimulated by psychoanalysis, but it can be speculated that the trend toward a subjective view of human failings might have occured without Freudian prodding. Cycles in scientific endeavor occur with the same inevitability that seems to guide the fate of empires and governments. The regularity that attends the circadian rhythm of the body also runs through nature, a pattern that seems predetermined in our universe. In the neural sciences to which psychiatry clings, the cycles of organicity vs. psychologism follow each other with a periodicity found in less subjective phenomena. Can it be that the mind of man is unable to sustain one direction or inquiry without succumbing to a fatigue factor induced by frustration in not coming upon the *real* truth?

From the position of the 1980s where neurophysiology and neurochemistry hold a favored scientific posture, the progress occurring early in the century may be regarded as quaint in the future. Perhaps biochemistry, electronic and sanitary engineering, and nutrition, will provide more advances in physical and mental health than have the innovations outlined herein. Still, every generation of workers enjoys its triumphs and suffers from its defeats. Clearly the task of understanding the functions and dysfunctions of the brain and mind is not completed, and it may never be. Nevertheless, the many whose efforts illuminated psychiatry in this node of time deserve to have their successes and struggles toward mental health recorded.

NOTES

1. Leo Kessel and Harold Hyman, "The Value of Psychoanalysis as a Therapeutic Procedure," *Journal of the American Medical Association* (hereafter *JAMA*) 101 (November 1933): 1612-15.

2. Harold Hyman, "The Value of Psychoanalysis as a Therapeutic Procedure," *JAMA* 107 (August 1936): 326-29.

3. Robert P. Knight, "Evaluation of the Results of Psychoanalytic Therapy," *American Journal of Psychiatry* 98 (November 1941): 434-46.

4. Hans Hoff, "The Invention of Insulin Shock Treatment of Schizophrenia, A Milestone in the Development of Psychiatry," in *Biologic Treatment of Mental Illness,* ed. M. Rinkel (New York: L. C. Page Co., 1966), p. 38.

5. J. F. Bateman and Nicholas Michael, "Pharmacologic Treatment of Schizophrenia," *American Journal of Psychiatry* 97 (July 1940): 59.

6. John R. Ross, et al., "The Pharmacologic Shock Treatment of Schizophrenia," *American Journal of Psychiatry* 97 (March 1941): 1007.

7. Lawrence Kolb and Victor Vogel, "The Use of Shock Treatment in 305 Mental Hospitals," *American Journal of Psychiatry* 99 (July 1942): 90-100.

8. See A. E. Bennett, "Curare: A Preventive of Traumatic Complications in Convulsive Shock Therapy," *American Journal of Psychiatry* 9 (March 1941): 1040-60; David J. Impastato, John Frosch, and S. Bernard Wortis, "Modifications of the Electro-fit," *American Journal of Psychiatry* 100 (November 1943): 358; Wilse G. Robinson, "The Treatment of Delirium with Insulin in Sub-shock Doses," *American Journal of Psychiatry* 97 (July 1940): 136; and Louis Wender, Ben Balser, and David Beres, "Extra-mural Shock Therapy," *American Journal of Psychiatry* 100 (March 1943): 712.

9. Richard M. Brickner, "The German Cultural Paranoid Trend," *American Journal of Orthopsychiatry* 12 (1942): 611-32.

10. Dorian Feigenbaum, "On Projection," *Psychoanalytic Quarterly* 5 (1936): 303-19.

11. Otto Fenichel, "Psychoanalysis of Anti-Semitism," *American Imago* 1 (1940): 24-39.

12. C. G. Jung, *The Integration of Personality* (New York: Farrar & Rhinehart, 1939).

13. M. Ralph Kaufman, Review, *Psychoanalytic Quarterly* 10 (1941): 652.

14. Edward Glover, *Freud or Jung* (New York: W. W. Norton, 1950), p. 152.

15. Carl G. Jung, *Man and his Symbols* (New York: Dell Pub. Co., 1964), p. 43.

16. Albert Deutsch, "Military Psychiatry, World War II," in *One Hundred Years of American Psychiatry,"* ed. American Psychiatric Association (New York: Columbia University Press, 1944), p. 420.

17. Dallas G. Sutton, "The Utilization of Psychiatry in the Armed Forces," *Psychiatry* 2, no. 1 (February 1939): 1.

18. Report, "Psychiatry and the National Defense," *Psychiatry* 3, no. 4 (November 1940): 619.

19. Comment, "Government Needs 600 Civilian Psychiatrists," *American Journal of Psychiatry* 97 (September 1940): 726.

20. Comment, "Psychiatry and the War," *American Journal of Psychiatry* 97 (January 1941): 972; Karl M. Menninger, Presidential Address, American Psychoanalytic Association, May, 1942," *Psychoanalytic Quarterly* 11 (1942): 299.

21. Wilfred Bloomberg and Robert Hyde, "A Survey of Neuropsychiatic Work at the Boston Induction Station," *American Journal of Psychiatry* 99 (July 1942): 23.

22. Alexander Simon and Margaret Hagan, "Social Data in Psychiatric Casualties in the Armed Services," *American Journal of Psychiatry* 99 (November 1942): 348.

23. Roy D. Halloran and Paul I. Yakolev, "Courses in Military Neuropsychiatry," *American Journal of Psychiatry* 99 (November 1942): 338.

24. Norman G. Brill, *Neuro-psychiatry in World War II*, vol. 1, (Washington D. C.: Office of the Surgeon General, Zone of the Interior, 1966), p. 195.

25. "Symposium on Military Psychiatry," *American Journal of Psychiatry* 100 (July 1943): 1-143.

26. Karl Menninger, "Presidential Address," p. 299.

27. Joseph Wortis, Karl M. Bowman, and Walter Goldfarb, "Human Brain Metabolisms," *American Journal of Psychiatry* 140 (November 1940): 552.

28. See Abraham Kardiner, *The Bio-Analysis of the Epileptic Reaction* (Albany, N.Y.: Psychoanalytic Press, 1932); Kardiner, *Traumatic Neurosis of War* (New York: Paul B. Hoeber, 1941).

29. Benjamin Apfelberg, "Experiences with the New Criminal Code in New York State," *American Journal of Psychiatry* 98 (November 1940): 415.

30. Walter Bromberg, "The Effects of War on Crime," *American Sociological Review* 8, no. 6 (December 1943): 685.

31. Special Committee to Secretary of War on Induction, *Neuropsychiatry in World War II*, vol. 1 (Washington D. C.: Office of Surgeon General, Zone of Interior, 1966), p. 805.

32. Winfred Overholser, "Review of Psychiatric Progress for 1941: Military Psychiatry," *American Journal of Psychiatry* 98 (January 1942): 581.

33. Deutsch, "Military Psychiatry, World War II," in *One Hundred Years of American Psychiatry*, p. 426.

34. Bernard Locke, et al., "Study of 1063 Naval Offenders," *U.S. Naval Bulletin* (1944): 73.

35. Walter Bromberg, Bernard Locke, and Anthony Apuzzo, "A Psychologic Study of Desertion and Overleave in the Navy," *U. S. Naval Bulletin* (1945): 558.

36. Samuel E. Morison, *The Oxford History of the American People* (New York: Oxford University Press, 1965), p. 1005.

37. Ibid., p. 1020.

38. Walter Bromberg, and Terry C. Rodgers, "Authority in the Treatment of Delinquents," *American Journal of Orthopsychiatry* 16 (October 1946): 672.

39. Walter Bromberg, "Dynamic Aspects of Psychopathic Personality," *Psychoanalytic Quarterly* 17 (January 1948): 58-70.

40. Carl Jonas, "Psychiatry Has Growing Pains," *American Journal of Psychiatry* 102 (1945): 819-24.

41. Roy R. Grinker and John P. Spiegel, *War Neuroses in North Africa* (Air Surgeon Army Air Force [Restricted]. New York: Josiah Macy Foundation, 1943).

42. Manfred Guttmacher and Frank A. Stewart, "A Psychiatric Study of Absence Without Leave," *American Journal of Psychiatry* 102 (July 1945): 74-81.

43. Lewis Loeser, "The Sexual Psychopath in Military Service," *American Journal of Psychiatry* 102 (July 1945): 92-101.

44. George C. Burns, "Neuropsychiatric Problems at an Aleutian Post," *American Journal of Psychiatry* 102 (1945): 205-13.

45. Bernard Diamond and Alice Ross, "Emotional Adjustment of Newly Blinded Soldiers," *American Journal of Psychiatry* 102 (1945): 367-71.

46. David Rothschild, "Review of Neuro-psychiatric Cases in the Southwest Pacific," *American Journal of Psychiatry* 102 (1945): 455-59.

47. Joseph L. Knapp and Frederick Weitzen, "A Total Psychotherapeutic Push Method as Practiced in the Fifth Service Command Rehabiliation Center, Fort Knox, Kentucky," *American Journal of Psychiatry* 102 (November 1945): 362-66.

48. Manfred Guttmacher, "Army Consultation Services," *American Journal of Psychiatry* 102 (May 1946): 735-48.

49. Harry C. Butcher, *My Three Years with Eisenhower* (New York: Simon & Schuster, 1946), p. 645.

50. Ibid., p. 390.

51. Jonas, "Psychiatry Has Growing Pains," p. 821.

52. Paul H. Hoch, "Review of Psychiatric Progress," *American Journal of Psychiatry* 102 (January 1946): 507-54.

BIBLIOGRAPHIC ESSAY

Psychiatric literature during the second, third, and fourth decades of this century experienced an enormous growth in books, monographs, and journal articles on mental and emotional troubles. This activity, however, was not limited to only the twentieth century. As judged by Henry Alden Bunker's comprehensive "American Psychiatric Literature During the Past Hundred Years," which appeared in the encyclopedic centenary volume put out by the American Psychiatric Association in 1944, there was no lack of papers in that earlier period. The present outline by no means covers the output of psychiatric material, even when it is confined to the 1918 to 1945 era.

At the turn of the century, textbooks originating in America, as Spitzka's *Insanity, Its Classification, Diagnosis and Treatment* (1883), chiefly followed the German and English masters—Henry Maudsley, Wilhelm Griesinger, and Emil Kraepelin. Translations of Kraepelin's *Lehrbuch der Psychiatrie* (1907) and Eugen Bleuler's *Textbook of Psychiatry* (1924) soon preempted the field until the appearance of Sir David Henderson and R. D. Gillespie's *A Textbook of Psychiatry for Students and Practitioners* (London, 1927), and by Edward A. Strecker and Franklin G. Ebaugh's *Practical Clinical Psychiatry* (Philadelphia, 1925). Henderson intended the text to present "psychiatry as a living subject . . . related to social problems of everyday life," and Strecker's book promulgated the "psychiatric viewpoint" to the medical profession. Although both these texts were influenced by Adolf Meyer's contributions, they represented the "modern" viewpoint with less accent on descriptive details.

It should be noted that the older texts, such as *Textbook of Nervous Diseases* by Charles L. Dana (1905) included discussions of nervous conditions— "a degenerate type of phrenasthenias [neurotics)"—in addition to strictly organic conditions. One of the earliest books to espouse the dynamic, that is Freudian contributions, was a neurological text *Diseases of the Nervous System* by Smith Ely Jelliffe and William A. White (1915), which was enlarged in 1923. It contained a long section on mental diseases, a tradition carried on in neurological texts as late as 1952 in Israel Wechsler's *Textbook of Clinical Neurology,* seventh edition.

One of the earliest dynamic treatments of psychiatry written was *Outline of Psychiatry* (1907) by William A. White, which remained a classic for years. Prior to the stimulus provided to psychiatric writings by psychoanalysis, such psychologists as Morton Prince, Boris Sidis, and J. J. Putnam were merging studies of double personalities and other mental abnormalities with psychological theories of perception, motivation, intellection in a way that exerted a tangential effect of clinical psychiatry. Thus Prince's *The Dissociation of a Personality* (1905), Sidis's *Foundations of Normal and Abnormal Psychology* (1914), and J. J. Putnam's *Human Motives* (1917) linked discussions of the subconscious with clinical and philosophic matters. Putnam, a neuropsychiatrist associated with Harvard exerted a strong influence and fostered Freudianism in American psychiatry.

Among the journals, the *American Journal of Psychiatry,* known as the *American Journal of Insanity* until 1921, continued the flood of papers that covered the whole gamut of clinical psychoses, the neuropathology of common psychoses, and discussions of epilepsy and syphilis, senility, and degenerative conditions. In the late 1920s the journal began to include studies spurred on by dynamic concepts. In consonance with the trend to consider the field united under the banner of neuropsychiatry, the *Archives of Neurology and Psychiatry* included many articles on psychiatric subjects until about 1930. Like the *American Journal of Psychiatry,* it served as a unifier for the profession by including book reviews, abstracts of European and native articles, society transactions, and notes of neuropsychiatric happenings. The *Journal of Nervous and Mental Disease,* chiefly a neurological publication in the nineteenth century, came under the editorship of Smith Ely Jelliffe after 1902. At the same time, the publication of the *Psychoanalytic Review* in 1913 by William Alanson White and Jelliffe constituted the first American publication devoted to psychoanalysis; it continued for many years under the unique leadership of Jelliffe.

The *Psychiatric Quarterly,* originally the *State Hospitals Bulletin* of the New York state hospital system, carried clinical articles from an early date to the present. The *Journal of the American Medical Association* also included occasional articles of general interest on psychiatry, general paresis (from 1900 to 1930), endocrinology, and development of therapies for mental and emotional conditions.

With the acceptance of psychoanalysis in this country, particularly in metropolitan centers, new journals appeared; *Psychiatry* emphasizing "the pathology of interpersonal relations," began in 1938; the *American Journal of Orthopsychiatry* in 1930; and the *Psychoanalytic Quarterly* in 1932. *Mental Hygiene* (1917), representing the national committee, focused on problems of the mental health movement's growth, including book reviews and notes, lay just on the periphery of clincial psychiatry and extended into psychiatric social work. This latter field, signaled by *The Kingdom of Evils* (1922) by Elmer E. Southard and Mary C. Jarrett, brought social problems and psychiatry into intimate relation. The *Psychoanalytic Quarterly,* probably the most influential journal in the 1930s and 1940s, started under the editorship of Dorian Feigenbaum, Bertram Lewin, Frankwood Williams, and Gregory Zilboorg and dedicated its first issue to the "need for a strictly psychoanalytic organ in America . . . [with] close collaboration of associates abroad." The *Journal of Criminal Psychopathology* (1939) featured articles on psychiatric criminology; the *Bulletin of the Menninger Clinic* (1936), *Psychosomatic Medicine* (1939), the *Quarterly Journal of Studies on Alcohol* (1940), and *The Nervous Child* (1941), all attested to the spread of psychiatric interests.

It would consume many pages to catalogue the books that were influential in the burgeoning field of psychiatry between the wars. Scientific and popular books poured off the presses in great numbers from 1930 on. Aside from translations of Freud's works from 1909 through 1920, the majority of which were done by A. A. Brill, books like Edward J. Kempf's *Psychopathology* (1920), William White's *Forty Years of Psychiatry* (1933), Sheldon and Eleanor Glueck's *One Thousand Juvenile Delinquents* (1934), Leo Kanner's *Child Psychiatry* (1935), Flanders Dunbar's *Emotion and Bodily Change* (1938), Karl A. Menninger's *Man Against Himself* (1938), and many others were the products of American authors. The spread of psychiatric preoccupation can be measured by such pioneer works as Abram Kardiner's *The Individual and his Society* (1939), an entrance into cultural and social psychiatry; *Science and Seizures* by William G. Lennox (1941), a study of epilepsy; David M. Levy's *Maternal Overprotection;* Gregory Zilboorg's *History of Medical Psychology* (1941); the present author's *Mind of Man,* a history of psychotherapy (1937); and Jules Masserman on *Behavior and Neurosis* (1943). Suffice it to say that fields of clinical psychiatry, organic states, child guidance, criminology, treatment methods, alcoholism, psychiatric social work, epilepsy, psychoanalysis, and personality problems attest to this wide spread of concern with human problems in health and disease.

The selection of significant or pioneering works during the period under discussion depends on the individual's judgment. Out of the welter of books, the later works of Freud, certainly *Civilization and Its Discontents,* written in 1927 and translated in 1930, his papers (1925 to

1938) collected in the fifth volume of *The Complete Psychological Works of Sigmund Freud* translated by James Strachey (1950) and containing such important papers as *Analysis Terminable and Interminable, Female Sexuality, Dostoevsky and Parricide,* should be mentioned. Other psychoanalytic works deserve mention: *The Psychoanalytic Theory of Neurosis* by Otto Fenichel (1945), Karen Horney's *Neurotic Personality of Our Time* (1937), and Erich Fromm's *Escape from Freedom* (1941). In clinical fields the textbook by Arthur Noyes, first published in 1934 and now grown to a comprehensive text entitled *Modern Clinical Psychiatry* under Lawrence Kolb (1981), was an outstanding American product. There were many authors whose final products were published after World War II and were based on work during the early 1940s. These included Harry S. Sullivan, Paul Schilder, Hervey Cleckley, Manfred Guttmacher, Walter Freeman, Franz Alexander, Lauretta Bender, Gregory Bateson, Frieda Fromm-Reichmann, Luther Kalinowsky, and many others. The clinical, laboratory, and therapeutic innovations of the 1918 to 1945 era flowered into a veritable Niagara of publications as the psychological disciplines attained their present growth after World War I.

Most of the secondary literature on psychiatry in the 1918 to 1945 period is found in restricted monographic contributions, for example in a number of papers published in the *Journal of the History of the Behavioral Sciences* and the history of medicine journals. These, along with many other items, are indexed in such standard guides as the *Bibliography of the History of Medicine.* Two recent collections of essays in particular serve to provide an opening into much of the extant historical writing: G. E. Gifford, ed., *Psychoanalysis, Psychotherapy, and the New England Medical Scene, 1894-1944* (1978) and Jacques Quen and Eric T. Carlson, eds., *American Psychoanalysis: Origins and Development* (1978). More systematic introductions can be found in George Mora and Jeanne Brand, eds., *Psychiatry and Its History, Methodological Problems in Research* (1970), and Daniel Blain and Michael Barton, *The History of American Psychiatry: A Teaching and Research Guide* (1979).

INDEX

About the Author

WALTER BROMBERG, a practicing neuro-psychiatrist and psychiatrist, is Adjunct Professor of Legal Medicine at the McGeorge School of Law, University of the Pacific, Sacramento, and a Consultant in Neurology and Psychiatry for the California State Department of Rehabilitation. A member of the American Psychiatric Association, Bromberg received his fifty years service award in May 1982. He is the author of several books on criminology, psychotherapy, and forensic psychiatry, including the classic *Mind of Man, Crime and the Mind, Mold of Murder*, and *The Uses of Psychiatry in the Law* (Greenwood Press, 1979).